Substance Use Disorders in Adult Critically Ill Patients

Kunal Karamchandani • Jon E. Grant
Editors

Substance Use Disorders in Adult Critically Ill Patients

Springer

Editors
Kunal Karamchandani
Department of Anesthesiology and Pain Management
The University of Texas Southwestern Med
Dallas, TX, USA

Jon E. Grant
Department of Psychiatry and Behavioral Neurosciences
University of Chicago
Chicago, IL, USA

ISBN 978-3-031-67068-8 ISBN 978-3-031-67069-5 (eBook)
https://doi.org/10.1007/978-3-031-67069-5

This Springer imprint is published by the registered company Springer Nature Switzerland AG
The registered company address is: Gewerbestrasse 11, 6330 Cham, Switzerland

Contents

Chapter 1
Epidemiology and Impact of Substance Use Disorders on the Intensive Care Unit

Jon E. Grant

Prevalence of Substance Use Disorders in the General Population

Both alcohol and drug use disorders are common and associated with significant morbidity and mortality [1–3]. In fact, the current prevalence rates of alcohol use disorder and drug use disorders in the general population of the United States are approximately 13.9% and 3.9%, respectively, based on the National Epidemiologic Survey on Alcohol and Related Conditions [4, 5]. The lifetime prevalence rates of alcohol use disorder and drug use disorders in the general population of the United States are approximately 29.1% and 9.9%, respectively [4, 5]. This roughly translates to one out of every ten adults in America having a current substance use disorder and one out of every three people having a substance use disorder in their lifetime. Past-year rates of nicotine dependence are found in 14.0% of the adult US population as well [6].

Diagnosing a Substance Use Disorder

Clinically, we make the diagnosis of a substance use disorder based on the following criteria set forth by the American Psychiatric Association's Diagnostic and Statistical Manual of Mental Disorders (DSM-5). To meet the criteria for substance use disorder, the person must meet at least two criteria within the same 12-month period [7]. The DSM-5 further allows clinicians to specify how severe or how much

J. E. Grant (✉)
Department of Psychiatry and Behavioral Neurosciences, University of Chicago, Chicago, IL, USA
e-mail: jongrant@uchicago.edu

K. Karamchandani, J. E. Grant (eds.), *Substance Use Disorders in Adult Critically Ill Patients*, https://doi.org/10.1007/978-3-031-67069-5_1

of a problem the substance use disorder is, depending on how many symptoms are identified. Two or three symptoms indicate a mild substance use disorder, four or five symptoms indicate a moderate substance use disorder, and six or more symptoms indicate a severe substance use disorder.

Substance Use Disorder Criteria (Adapted from the DSM-5) [7]

The clinician using these criteria should first make sure a specific time period is being referenced. That is, does the patient endorse these symptoms within the past 12 months (i.e., a current problem) or ever during their lifetime? These criteria should be used separately for each substance that the person reports using. For example, all 11 symptoms should be examined for alcohol and then separately for cocaine, etc. The result of this assessment is that a person could have several substance use disorders, such as alcohol use disorder, cocaine use disorder, etc. As each substance necessitates different interventions, it is important to diagnose which substance use disorders the person has.

1. The person takes the substance in larger amounts or for longer than intended.
2. They try unsuccessfully to cut down on or stop using the substance.
3. They spend a lot of time trying to acquire, use, or recover from the substance.
4. The person reports cravings and urges to use the substance.
5. They fail to fulfill obligations at work, home, or school because of substance use.
6. Even when substance use results in relationship problems, they continue to use it.
7. They abandon important social, occupational, or recreational activities because of substance use.
8. They use the substance even when it puts them in danger.
9. Even when you know you have a physical or psychological problem that could have been caused or made worse by the substance, they continue to use it.
10. The amount of the substance increases over time to get the desired effect.
11. They experience withdrawal symptoms.

The DSM-5 criteria for substance use disorders is the gold standard, but many research reports and clinical settings may prefer to screen for alcohol and drug use disorders with shorter measures and then have mental health professionals do a follow-up assessment for any patient with a positive substance use disorder screen.

Prevalence of Substance Use Disorders in Medical Settings

As common as these problems are in the general population, data show that the rates of substance use disorders are even more frequently found in medical populations. In primary care settings, 20–30% of patients can be expected to have some current level of problem use of alcohol, and approximately 5–10% of patients have a current substance use disorder [8–10]. In hospital settings, the problems with substances are generally higher, with rates of current alcohol use disorder ranging as high as 19–50% and rates of current drug use disorders ranging from 12% to 15% [11–14].

Screening for Substance Use Disorders in Medical Settings

Because rates of substance use disorders are higher in medical settings compared to the overall population, screening for use problems should be considered in all hospital settings, including the emergency department and the intensive care units. Emergency room screening is recommended by the American College of Emergency Physicians, and as this may be the point of contact before the patient is admitted to an intensive care unit (ICU), the screening in the emergency department may assist with more appropriate treatment planning in the ICU. Ideally, a positive screen should be followed by a more detailed diagnostic assessment by trained mental health staff.

On a practical level, there are several measures that could be used in hospital settings, including the ICU, to screen for substance use problems. A couple of the most commonly reported instruments that are easy to use in an ICU to screen for alcohol and drug use in adults are the AUDIT and the DSAT-10. The Alcohol Use Disorders Identification Test (AUDIT) [15] is perhaps the most widely used screening tool for alcohol use. Instead of only screening for a formal alcohol use disorder, the measure screens for unhealthy use and provides a level of risk that the person meets (a score of ≥8 also suggests an alcohol use disorder). The most-used version has ten items and takes a couple of minutes to administer. In terms of screening for unhealthy drug use (or a substance use disorder), the most widely used measure is the Drug Abuse Screening Test (DSAT-10) [16]. It also consists of ten questions and takes only a few minutes to administer (a score of ≥3 also suggests a substance use disorder).

Screening in a hospital setting, such as an emergency department or ICU, is likely to result in a higher proportion of patients who screen positive, identify more severe substance use, and be associated with complex psychiatric and medical comorbidities compared to outpatient settings. Of course, screens are not the same as diagnostic measures, and they are intended to over-identify problems. Clinicians need to be aware of the limitations of these instruments and follow-up positive screens with more detailed assessments.

The goals of screening in the ICU, for example, will also differ from those in outpatient settings. At minimum, ICUs should screen to identify patients at high risk for acute withdrawal or for procedural complications related to their substance use. Screening in the ICU can also identify patients with substance use disorders who need medications or ongoing treatment post-discharge. When substance use disorders are identified by screening, ICUs may also afford themselves, where available, of addiction consult services, which typically involve a team-based approach to managing patients in the hospital and engaging them in post-discharge treatment and harm reduction services. Controlling the substance use disorder post-discharge is more likely to ensure the patient will also follow up with post-discharge medical care for whatever complex health problem was the reason for the ICU admission. This in turn should reduce readmission for the same problem or for complications.

Substance Use Disorders in the Intensive Care Unit

The epidemiology of substance use disorders in ICUs is largely unknown. As emergency departments tend to have higher rates of substance use disorders than in the general population, we might expect rates to be higher in ICUs as well, and some data support this heuristic. Using 2016–2017 emergency department data from the National Hospital Ambulatory Medical Care Survey, Zhang and colleagues examined adults with and without a substance use disorder and found that people seen in emergency departments who had substance use disorders were more likely to be hospitalized and admitted to the ICU (they were also more likely to experience homelessness, suffer from mental illness, and require ambulance services) [17]. One study reported that approximately 16–31% of patients in ICUs have an alcohol use disorder [18], which is higher than the current rate of 13.9% in the general population [4]. Estimates from one community hospital, however, reported that 14% of ICU admissions were non-tobacco substance-related [19], a rate similar to the general population [4]. Another study found that 19% of ICU admissions in New York City were due to alcohol and drug intoxication [20]. This study did not report rates of substance use disorders but instead examined any level of unhealthy alcohol or drug use. Another study found that of their mechanically ventilated patients in the ICU, 39% had a substance use disorder [21].

Based on the available research, ICUs constitute a setting where clinicians will have to be aware of and willing to manage a range of problems associated with substance use disorders as well as misuse of alcohol and drugs (i.e., use that may not be at the level of a substance use disorder but necessitates medical attention due to the health consequences of the substance use).

Not All Substance Use Is a Substance Use Disorder

Of course, not all alcohol and drug use meets the diagnostic criteria for a substance use disorder, and yet it can still impact patient care and outcomes. In fact, the screens mentioned above were created to also examine levels of use that might be below the severity of a substance use disorder but may still necessitate interventions as this can cause some problems for the person. Thus, there are gradients of use from no use to non-harmful recreational use, to misuse of drugs or alcohol (this might mean meeting a single criterion for a substance use disorder such as in the case of hazardous alcohol use), and finally to meeting DSM-5 diagnostic criteria for a substance use disorder (see above). In an ICU setting, this lower level of substance misuse will often result in the same acute interventions. The difference between misuse and a substance use disorder is generally more important for post-discharge treatment planning.

Even at lower levels of use (often referred to as misuse or hazardous use), however, alcohol and drugs can lead to ICU admissions and resultant health problems. Research suggests that prevalence rates of alcohol and drug misuse are actually higher than the rates of substance use disorders, but oftentimes only come to the attention of medical professionals when severe health problems occur [22–24]. For example, hazardous drinking is common among college students in the United States, with studies documenting prevalence estimates ranging from 33% to 57% [25]. A Finnish study of 2045 patients admitted to the ICU found that 21% screened positive for hazardous alcohol use [26]. Similarly, a trend worldwide has seen an increase in opiate misuse among people who in turn need ICU admissions [27], often leading to high mortality rates (up to 10%) [28].

Medical Problems Associated with Substance Use in the Intensive Care Unit

Beyond the range of long-term health issues associated with substance use disorders [29, 30], doctor and nurses in the ICU will often be called upon to manage substance intoxication and potential withdrawal in many people, even those who do not meet criteria for a use disorder. Additionally, as each substance results in different clinical manifestations of intoxication and withdrawal, staff in an ICU need to understand the clinical presentation of intoxication and withdrawal across a range of substances (the various chapters of this volume will present the unique issues related to each substance and management strategies).

One study suggested that approximately 16–31% of patients in an ICU are at risk for developing alcohol withdrawal syndrome, and this is likely the most common substance seen in ICU admissions [18]. Patients admitted to the ICU with alcohol withdrawal tend to have longer ICU stays, a longer duration of mechanical ventilation, higher costs, and increased mortality compared with those admitted who do not go through alcohol withdrawal [18].

Medical management of substance use disorders is not confined to the intoxication or withdrawal from the misused substance. There are substantial health comorbidities related to chronic drug and alcohol misuse that often need to be managed in the ICU, such as gastrointestinal bleeding due to alcohol misuse. Available data demonstrate that substance use problems are major risk factors associated with poor ICU outcomes. Patients in the ICU are more likely to experience delirium, which in turn complicates the management of comorbid health conditions [31]. In a large (n = 11,651) study of adult admissions to two urban ICUs, the researchers found that 12.2% had a diagnosis consistent with alcohol dependence, and those patients had higher rates of sepsis, organ failure, septic shock, and hospital mortality (a two-fold increased risk) [32].

Mental Health Problems Associated with Substance Use in the Intensive Care Unit

Because substance use disorders are highly comorbid with multiple psychiatric disorders [33], medical management of the substance problem in the ICU will further require the management of an array of mental health problems as well.

Rates of depression, anxiety, personality disorders, suicidality, psychosis, and bipolar disorder are all elevated in people who struggle with substance use disorder compared to the general community [34, 35] and may present unique challenges to the staff in the ICU. Although a detailed assessment and treatment plan for these comorbid psychiatric disorders will be presented in a later chapter, suffice it to say that consultation with mental health providers is often necessary during the ICU stay.

Costs of Substance Problems in the Intensive Care Unit

Substance problems in the ICU are costly to the healthcare system, but determining how costly is not always clear or easily done. An early 1993 study reported that 28% of ICU admissions over a 15-week period at Johns Hopkins Hospital were related to substance abuse and accrued 39% of the hospital costs for that period [36]. A more recent study of 611 ICU admissions over a 6-month period found that 25.7% of admissions were related to substance abuse and accrued 23.1% of total hospital charges, and more specifically, illicit drug-related admissions accounted for 13.1% of admissions associated with 11.1% of total hospital charges, while alcohol accounted for 9.7% of admissions and represented 7.8% of total charges [37]. In 2006, the estimated hospital costs for treatment of alcohol-related issues exceeded $5 billion, but the total estimated economic cost of excessive drinking exceeded $220 billion [38]. Another study found that in a 6-month period, alcohol and drug abuse patients accrued over 7 million US dollars, largely in ICU admissions, and that over 50% of this cohort were either admitted to Medicaid/managed care or obtained emergency Medicaid in hospital [20].

Even patients who do not have a substance use disorder but simply misuse alcohol or drugs still seem to increase healthcare costs. In a study examining several thousand patients in a national quality registry database for ICUs, the authors found that intoxicated patients admitted to the ICU had in the year before and after ICU admission much higher median healthcare costs per day compared to other ICU patients and a general population control group [39]. Several studies from hospitals around the world have found that the annual costs of drug and alcohol intoxication cost, on average, several million dollars per year per hospital [40–42].

Treatment in the ICU

Hospital-based addiction treatment can dramatically improve the health outcomes of hospitalized patients with substance use disorders and should begin in the ICU. Treatment for the various substance problems will be the focus of chapters within this volume. The vast majority of individuals with substance use disorders do not feel that they need treatment, with only 12.5% of people with substance use disorders perceiving a need for treatment [43]. In trauma patients, a formal discussion with their medical providers about their alcohol use, screening for alcohol problems, and a discussion of how their alcohol use contributed to their injury has been shown to significantly decrease recidivism in these patients for traumatic injuries associated with alcohol use. The acuity and direct correlation of the two problems (alcohol use and their injury) have been hypothesized to be a "teachable moment" with a greater chance of initiating change. Substance misuse that leads to an ICU admission is therefore an opportunity for medical providers to use the life-threatening medical problem to help patients with substance problems recognize the issue, which may be an impetus for seeking treatment or behavioral change.

Treatment After the ICU

Although chapters in this book will discuss post-discharge planning, it is important to note that discharge planning protocols, including medication-assisted treatment, for patients admitted with substance problems may reduce subsequent emergency room visits and 30-day rehospitalization. The addition of pharmacotherapy to psychosocial treatment in patients with alcohol problems has been shown to improve outcomes. Similarly, in patients admitted with opioid misuse, in-patient initiation of opioid agonist therapy and early discharge planning may reduce rates of AMA discharge and increase the likelihood of transfer to long-term out-patient addiction treatment.

Acknowledgment of Assistance None.

Previous Presentation None.

Relevant Financial Relationships Dr. Grant has received research grant support from NIDA, Biohaven, and Janssen Pharmaceuticals. He receives yearly compensation from Springer Publishing for acting as Editor-in-Chief of the Journal of Gambling Studies and has received royalties from Oxford University Press, American Psychiatric Publishing, Inc., Norton Press, and McGraw Hill.

References

1. Esser MB, Sherk A, Liu Y, Naimi TS, Stockwell T, Stahre M, Kanny D, Landen M, Saitz R, Brewer RD. Deaths and years of potential life lost from excessive alcohol use—United States, 2011–2015. MMWR Morb Mortal Wkly Rep. 2020;69(39):1428–33. https://doi.org/10.15585/mmwr.mm6939a6. PMID: 33001874; PMCID: PMC7537556.
2. Hedegaard H, Miniño AM, Warner M. Drug overdose deaths in the United States, 1999–2018. NCHS Data Brief. 2020;356:1–8.
3. Scott CK, Dennis ML, Laudet A, Funk RR, Simeone RS. Surviving drug addiction: the effect of treatment and abstinence on mortality. Am J Public Health. 2011;101(4):737–44. https://doi.org/10.2105/AJPH.2010.197038. Epub 2011 Feb 17. PMID: 21330586; PMCID: PMC3052346.
4. Grant BF, Goldstein RB, Saha TD, Chou SP, Jung J, Zhang H, Pickering RP, Ruan WJ, Smith SM, Huang B, Hasin DS. Epidemiology of DSM-5 alcohol use disorder: results from the National Epidemiologic Survey on Alcohol and Related Conditions III. JAMA Psychiatry. 2015;72(8):757–66. https://doi.org/10.1001/jamapsychiatry.2015.0584. PMID: 26039070; PMCID: PMC5240584.
5. Grant BF, Saha TD, Ruan WJ, Goldstein RB, Chou SP, Jung J, Zhang H, Smith SM, Pickering RP, Huang B, Hasin DS. Epidemiology of DSM-5 drug use disorder: results from the National Epidemiologic Survey on Alcohol and Related Conditions-III. JAMA Psychiatry. 2016;73(1):39–47. https://doi.org/10.1001/jamapsychiatry.2015.2132. PMID: 26580136; PMCID: PMC5062605.
6. Grant BF, Shmulewitz D, Compton WM. Nicotine use and DSM-IV nicotine dependence in the United States, 2001–2002 and 2012–2013. Am J Psychiatry. 2020;177(11):1082–90. https://doi.org/10.1176/appi.ajp.2020.19090900. Epub 2020 Aug 14.
7. American Psychiatric Association. Diagnostic and statistical manual of mental disorders. 5th ed. Washington, DC: American Psychiatric Association; 2013.
8. McNeely J, Hamilton L. Screening for unhealthy alcohol and drug use in general medicine settings. Med Clin North Am. 2022;106(1):13–28. https://doi.org/10.1016/j.mcna.2021.08.002.
9. Vinson DC, Manning BK, Galliher JM, Dickinson LM, Pace WD, Turner BJ. Alcohol and sleep problems in primary care patients: a report from the AAFP National Research Network. Ann Fam Med. 2010;8(6):484–92. https://doi.org/10.1370/afm.1175. PMID: 21060117; PMCID: PMC2975682.
10. Cherpitel CJ, Ye Y. Drug use and problem drinking associated with primary care and emergency room utilization in the US general population: data from the 2005 national alcohol survey. Drug Alcohol Depend. 2008;97(3):226–30. https://doi.org/10.1016/j.drugalcdep.2008.03.033. Epub 2008 May 21. PMID: 18499355; PMCID: PMC3007592.
11. Serowik KL, Yonkers KA, Gilstad-Hayden K, Forray A, Zimbrean P, Martino S. Substance use disorder detection rates among providers of general medical inpatients. J Gen Intern Med. 2021;36(3):668–75. https://doi.org/10.1007/s11606-020-06319-7. Epub 2020 Oct 27. PMID: 33111239; PMCID: PMC7947066.
12. Walley AY, Paasche-Orlow M, Lee EC, Forsythe S, Chetty VK, Mitchell S, Jack BW. Acute care hospital utilization among medical inpatients discharged with a substance use disorder diagnosis. J Addict Med. 2012;6(1):50–6. https://doi.org/10.1097/ADM.0b013e318231de51. PMID: 21979821; PMCID: PMC6034987.
13. Saitz R, Freedner N, Palfai TP, Horton NJ, Samet JH. The severity of unhealthy alcohol use in hospitalized medical patients. The spectrum is narrow. J Gen Intern Med. 2006;21(4):381–5. https://doi.org/10.1111/j.1525-1497.2006.00405.x. PMID: 16686818; PMCID: PMC1484710.
14. Smothers BA, Yahr HT. Alcohol use disorder and illicit drug use in admissions to general hospitals in the United States. Am J Addict. 2005;14(3):256–67. https://doi.org/10.1080/10550490590949433.
15. Saunders JB, Aasland OG, Babor TF, de la Fuente JR, Grant M. Development of the Alcohol Use Disorders Identification Test (AUDIT): WHO collaborative project on early detection of

persons with harmful alcohol consumption--II. Addiction. 1993;88(6):791–804. https://doi.org/10.1111/j.1360-0443.1993.tb02093.x.
16. Skinner HA. The drug abuse screening test. Addict Behav. 1982;7(4):363–71. https://doi.org/10.1016/0306-4603(82)90005-3.
17. Zhang X, Wang N, Hou F, Ali Y, Dora-Laskey A, Dahlem CH, McCabe SE. Emergency department visits by patients with substance use disorder in the United States. West J Emerg Med. 2021;22(5):1076–85. https://doi.org/10.5811/westjem.2021.3.50839. PMID: 34546883; PMCID: PMC8463055.
18. Dixit D, Endicott J, Burry L, Ramos L, Yeung SY, Devabhakthuni S, Chan C, Tobia A, Bulloch MN. Management of acute alcohol withdrawal syndrome in critically ill patients. Pharmacotherapy. 2016;36(7):797–822. https://doi.org/10.1002/phar.1770. Epub 2016 Jun 30.
19. Donroe JH, Tetrault JM. Substance use, intoxication, and withdrawal in the critical care setting. Crit Care Clin. 2017;33(3):543–58. https://doi.org/10.1016/j.ccc.2017.03.003. Epub 2017 Apr 20.
20. Cervellione KL, Shah A, Patel MC, Curiel Duran L, Ullah T, Thurm C. Alcohol and drug abuse resource utilization in the ICU. Subst Abuse. 2019;13:1178221819869327. https://doi.org/10.1177/1178221819869327. PMID: 31548794; PMCID: PMC6743197.
21. de Wit M, Wan SY, Gill S, Jenvey WI, Best AM, Tomlinson J, Weaver MF. Prevalence and impact of alcohol and other drug use disorders on sedation and mechanical ventilation: a retrospective study. BMC Anesthesiol. 2007;7:3. https://doi.org/10.1186/1471-2253-7-3. PMID: 17359534; PMCID: PMC1838409.
22. DiGuiseppi C, Goss C, Xu S, Magid D, Graham A. Telephone screening for hazardous drinking among injured patients seen in acute care clinics: feasibility study. Alcohol Alcohol. 2006;41(4):438–45. https://doi.org/10.1093/alcalc/agl031. Epub 2006 May 5.
23. Moe J, Camargo CA, Jelinski S, Erdelyi S, Brubacher J, Rowe BH. Epidemiologic trends in substance and opioid misuse-related emergency department visits in Alberta: a cross-sectional time-series analysis. Can J Public Health. 2018;109(2):164–73. https://doi.org/10.17269/s41997-018-0053-6. Epub 2018 May 9. PMID: 29981040; PMCID: PMC6964387.
24. Bachhuber MA, Maughan BC, Mitra N, Feingold J, Starrels JL. Prescription monitoring programs and emergency department visits involving benzodiazepine misuse: early evidence from 11 United States metropolitan areas. Int J Drug Policy. 2016;28:120–3. https://doi.org/10.1016/j.drugpo.2015.08.005. Epub 2015 Aug 13. PMID: 26345658; PMCID: PMC4752854.
25. Paulus DJ, Zvolensky MJ. The prevalence and impact of elevated anxiety sensitivity among hazardous drinking college students. Drug Alcohol Depend. 2020;209:107922. https://doi.org/10.1016/j.drugalcdep.2020.107922. Epub 2020 Feb 15. PMID: 32088590; PMCID: PMC7536785.
26. Nissilä E, Hynninen M, Reinikainen M, Bendel S, Suojaranta R, Korhonen AM, Suvela M, Loisa P, Kaminski T, Hästbacka J. Prevalence and impact of hazardous alcohol use in intensive care cohort: a multicenter, register-based study. Acta Anaesthesiol Scand. 2021;65(8):1073–8. https://doi.org/10.1111/aas.13828. Epub 2021 Jul 27.
27. Friebel R, Maynou L. Trends and characteristics of hospitalisations from the harmful use of opioids in England between 2008 and 2018: population-based retrospective cohort study. J R Soc Med. 2022;115(5):173–85. https://doi.org/10.1177/01410768221077360. Epub 2022 Feb 3. PMID: 35114090; PMCID: PMC9066666.
28. Pfister GJ, Burkes RM, Guinn B, Steele J, Kelley RR, Wiemken TL, Saad M, Ramirez J, Cavallazzi R. Opioid overdose leading to intensive care unit admission: epidemiology and outcomes. J Crit Care. 2016;35:29–32. https://doi.org/10.1016/j.jcrc.2016.04.022. Epub 2016 Apr 30.
29. Simet SM, Sisson JH. Alcohol's effects on lung health and immunity. Alcohol Res. 2015;37(2):199–208. PMID: 26695745; PMCID: PMC4590617.
30. Quaglio G, Lugoboni F, Pattaro C, GICS, Montanari L, Lechi A, Mezzelani P, Des Jarlais DC. Patients in long-term maintenance therapy for drug use in Italy: analysis of some param-

eters of social integration and serological status for infectious diseases in a cohort of 1091 patients. BMC Public Health. 2006;6:216. https://doi.org/10.1186/1471-2458-6-216. PMID: 16928267; PMCID: PMC1570141.
31. Steel TL, Bhatraju EP, Hills-Dunlap K. Critical care for patients with substance use disorders. Curr Opin Crit Care. 2023;29(5):484–92. https://doi.org/10.1097/MCC.0000000000001080. Epub 2023 Jul 31.
32. O'Brien JM Jr, Lu B, Ali NA, Martin GS, Aberegg SK, Marsh CB, Lemeshow S, Douglas IS. Alcohol dependence is independently associated with sepsis, septic shock, and hospital mortality among adult intensive care unit patients. Crit Care Med. 2007;35(2):345–50. https://doi.org/10.1097/01.CCM.0000254340.91644.B2.
33. Hasin D, Kilcoyne B. Comorbidity of psychiatric and substance use disorders in the United States: current issues and findings from the NESARC. Curr Opin Psychiatry. 2012;25(3):165–71. https://doi.org/10.1097/YCO.0b013e3283523dcc. PMID: 22449770; PMCID: PMC3767413.
34. Grant BF, Stinson FS, Dawson DA, Chou SP, Dufour MC, Compton W, Pickering RP, Kaplan K. Prevalence and co-occurrence of substance use disorders and independent mood and anxiety disorders: results from the National Epidemiologic Survey on Alcohol and Related Conditions. Arch Gen Psychiatry. 2004;61(8):807–16. https://doi.org/10.1001/archpsyc.61.8.807.
35. Trull TJ, Jahng S, Tomko RL, Wood PK, Sher KJ. Revised NESARC personality disorder diagnoses: gender, prevalence, and comorbidity with substance dependence disorders. J Personal Disord. 2010;24(4):412–26. https://doi.org/10.1521/pedi.2010.24.4.412. PMID: 20695803; PMCID: PMC3771514.
36. Baldwin WA, Rosenfeld BA, Breslow MJ, Buchman TG, Deutschman CS, Moore RD. Substance abuse-related admissions to adult intensive care. Chest. 1993;103(1):21–5. https://doi.org/10.1378/chest.103.1.21.
37. Westerhausen D, Perkins AJ, Conley J, Khan BA, Farber M. Burden of substance abuse-related admissions to the medical ICU. Chest. 2020;157(1):61–6. https://doi.org/10.1016/j.chest.2019.08.2180. Epub 2019 Sep 5.
38. Colling K, Kraft AK, Harry ML. Alcohol use disorder in the intensive care unit a highly morbid condition, but chemical dependency discussion improves outcomes. Acute Crit Care. 2023;38(1):122–33. https://doi.org/10.4266/acc.2022.00584. Epub 2023 Jan 10. PMID: 36935541; PMCID: PMC10030241.
39. van Beusekom I, Bakhshi-Raiez F, de Keizer NF, de Lange DW. The healthcare costs of intoxicated patients who survive ICU admission are higher than non-intoxicated ICU patients: a retrospective study combining healthcare insurance data and data from a Dutch national quality registry. BMC Emerg Med. 2019;19(1):6. https://doi.org/10.1186/s12873-019-0224-7. PMID: 30634921; PMCID: PMC6329083.
40. Welch C, Harrison D, Short A, Rowan K. The increasing burden of alcoholic liver disease on United Kingdom critical care units: secondary analysis of a high quality clinical database. J Health Serv Res Policy. 2008;13(Suppl 2):40–4. https://doi.org/10.1258/jhsrp.2007.007101.
41. Geary T, O'Brien P, Ramsay S, Cook B, Scottish Intensive Care Trainees' Audit Share Group. A national service evaluation of the impact of alcohol on admissions to Scottish intensive care units. Anaesthesia. 2012;67(10):1132–7. https://doi.org/10.1111/j.1365-2044.2012.07233.x. Epub 2012 Jul 16.
42. McMahon A, Brohan J, Donnelly M, Fitzpatrick GJ. Characteristics of patients admitted to the intensive care unit following self-poisoning and their impact on resource utilisation. Ir J Med Sci. 2014;183(3):391–5. https://doi.org/10.1007/s11845-013-1026-7. Epub 2013 Oct 8.
43. Moeller SJ, Platt JM, Wu M, Goodwin RD. Perception of treatment need among adults with substance use disorders: longitudinal data from a representative sample of adults in the United States. Drug Alcohol Depend. 2020;209:107895. https://doi.org/10.1016/j.drugalcdep.2020.107895. Epub 2020 Feb 6. PMID: 32078975; PMCID: PMC7418940.

Chapter 2
Alcohol Abuse Disorder: Alcohol Withdrawal Syndrome

Deepali Dixit, Marissa Grillo, Jessica Hu, and Maria Cardinale-King

Introduction

Alcohol use disorder is a prevalent issue, affecting around 28.6 million adults, and is especially common among those who are hospitalized [1, 2]. Patients with alcohol use disorder are at risk for alcohol withdrawal syndrome (AWS), which may require admission to the intensive care unit (ICU) [3]. AWS poses significant challenges in the ICU due to its potential for severe complications. Patients admitted to the ICU with AWS have a higher mortality rate, longer ICU stays, a longer duration of ventilator support, and higher costs compared with patients without AWS [4, 5]. A substantial proportion of ICU admissions are related to alcohol abuse. The incidence of AWS in the ICU varies, but estimates range from 20% to 30% of patients with alcohol dependence [2, 3]. AWS encompasses a spectrum of symptoms that develop after either sudden cessation or abrupt reduction of alcohol intake in long-term alcohol users [6]. Symptoms can range from mild, such as anxiety and tremors, to severe or fatal, including delirium tremens (DTs) and seizures, which occur in approximately 20% of patients admitted to the hospital with AWS [7, 8]. AWS is associated with up to 10% of annual Medical ICU (MICU) admissions [9], and the burden associated with this diagnosis exceeds 250 billion US dollars annually [10].

One of the goals of AWS treatment is to prevent the occurrence of the most severe symptoms in high-risk patients. Early identification and treatment are vital in reducing the risk of progressing to severe AWS [11]. Unfortunately, this history can be difficult to obtain for critically ill patients who may not be able to communicate

D. Dixit (✉) · J. Hu · M. Cardinale-King
Ernest Mario School of Pharmacy, Rutgers, The State University of New Jersey, Piscataway, NJ, USA
e-mail: ddixit@pharmacy.rutgers.edu

M. Grillo
Hackensack University Medical Center, Hackensack, NJ, USA

K. Karamchandani, J. E. Grant (eds.), *Substance Use Disorders in Adult Critically Ill Patients*, https://doi.org/10.1007/978-3-031-67069-5_2

and who may not have a proxy to provide the information. Patients with a history of prior withdrawal, seizures, or DTs, or those consuming alcohol while being treated for alcohol use disorder, are at a greater risk for withdrawal [3].

With advancements in medical care and pharmacotherapy options, most patients survive AWS acutely [12]. However, many patients remain at risk after the acute AWS episode has subsided because of alcohol use after discharge. Approximately 44% of ICU patients who survive AWS are rehospitalized at least once or experience death within a year [13].

Pathophysiology of AWS

The pathophysiology of AWS involves several interconnected mechanisms, and some of the key aspects are described here. Ethanol's primary action on the central nervous system (CNS) is mediated by the disruption of two major neurotransmitter pathways: the inhibitory neurotransmitter gamma-aminobutyric acid (GABA) and the excitatory neurotransmitter glutamate, which binds to the N-methyl-D-aspartate (NMDA) receptor [5, 14].

1. Neuroadaptation: Chronic alcohol use leads to neuroadaptation, where the brain adjusts its functioning to compensate for the presence of alcohol. The brain becomes more excitable, and the GABA receptors are upregulated to counteract alcohol's sedating effects.
2. GABAergic and Glutamatergic Systems: With the sudden cessation of alcohol, the upregulated GABA system continues to function, causing an imbalance between inhibitory and excitatory neurotransmitters. The chronic suppression of the excitatory neurotransmitter glutamate due to alcohol's inhibitory effects is suddenly unopposed, leading to hyperexcitability.
3. Excitatory Hyperactivity: The unopposed glutamate activity triggers excitatory hyperactivity, resulting in symptoms such as anxiety, restlessness, tremors, and seizures. This hyperactivity can also contribute to increased sympathetic nervous system activity, leading to elevated heart rate, blood pressure, and diaphoresis.
4. Withdrawal Seizures: Alcohol withdrawal seizures are thought to result from hyperexcitability in the brain, primarily involving the limbic system and the kindling effect. Kindling refers to the phenomenon where repeated alcohol withdrawals lead to an increased risk and severity of subsequent seizures.
5. Alcohol Withdrawal Delirium (Delirium Tremens): In severe cases, AWS can progress to delirium tremens (DTs). The exact mechanisms behind DTs are not fully understood, but they involve complex interactions between neurotransmitters, neuroinflammation, and imbalances in the brain's reward system. DTs are characterized by severe confusion, hallucinations, and cardiovascular instability and can be life-threatening.

Table 2.1 Stages of alcohol withdrawal symptoms [3, 15, 16]

Stage	Time since the last alcoholic drink	Signs and symptoms
1	6–24 hours	Tremor Autonomic activity Insomnia/agitation Tachypnea/hyperventilation Headache Sweating Anorexia/nausea/vomiting
2	7–48 hours	Distractibility, tonic-clonic seizures (10% of patients) Visual, tactile, or auditory hallucinations (30% of patients) Autonomic instability Diarrhea
3	49–96 hours	Intense tremor ➔ delirium tremens (5% of patients [25% mortality].) Severe autonomic instability Confusion/disorientation/extreme agitation

Clinical Presentation

AWS represents a continuous spectrum of symptoms, ranging from mild symptoms to DTs. The clinical presentation of AWS is individualized and influenced by the patient's intake pattern, comorbidities, and genetics [11]. While some patients may not exhibit any symptoms, others may experience mild ones like insomnia, and some may even develop severe AWS, which can include DTs [11]. The signs and symptoms of AWS are well-defined. It is believed that they occur in stages, although not every patient experiences a symptom in each stage. (Table 2.1) [15]. DTs are the longest-lasting symptom of AWS and may occur as long as ten days after the onset of AWS and may last for up to five days [15]. They are more likely to occur in patients with a history of DTs and those who have low albumin levels, are hypotensive, are tachycardic, have a high blood urea nitrogen level, or have a coexisting medical illness [15]. DTs are a rare, serious complication of AWS associated with disorientation and profound autonomic symptoms such as tachycardia, severe agitation, fever, and hypertension [15].

Screening Tools

Symptom-triggered benzodiazepine protocols are the standard of care for the treatment of AWS [16] because they have been shown to reduce benzodiazepine use and total treatment time compared to fixed-dose protocols [17, 18]. The Clinical Institute of Withdrawal Assessment for Alcohol, revised (CIWA-Ar), is the most common symptom-triggered assessment tool [19]. However, the CIWA-Ar is a ten-item instrument and relies on many subjective symptoms (e.g., anxiety, headache, nausea); therefore, shorter and more objective scales may be helpful. Nine of the ten CIWA-Ar items are scored using a broad 0–7 scale, raising concern for interrater variability. Moreover, because of the subjective items, CIWA-Ar cannot be used on patients who are delirious or cannot communicate. Once AWS occurs, early and frequent assessment of symptoms is necessary to avoid potential complications such as seizures. Several withdrawal and objective sedation-agitation scales have been used to rate the severity of symptoms in patients experiencing AWS. The revised CIWA-Ar and the Riker Sedation-Agitation Scale (SAS) are the most frequently used tools for this purpose. Based on the available evidence, combining the use of the CIWA-Ar tool in patients capable of communication and SAS to titrate benzodiazepines for agitation symptoms in ICU patients that are unable to communicate may be the best approach to match medication dosing with symptom severity to improve outcomes. The Richmond Agitation-Sedation Scale (RASS) has also been used to titrate benzodiazepines and other agents in patients with severe AWS, including those requiring mechanical ventilation [20].

Supportive Care

Clinicians must be aware of the complications that can develop in a patient during withdrawal to provide appropriate management. The goals of care are to alleviate AWS symptoms, prevent symptom progression, and treat underlying comorbidities. Adequate fluid resuscitation is particularly vital, as individuals with a history of alcoholism frequently experience intravascular depletion [5, 14]. Electrolyte deficiencies are common in this population and require vigilant monitoring and replacement [5, 14, 15]. Correcting these abnormalities may take several days of supplementation, depending on the patient's intracellular depletion. Electrolyte levels should be monitored at least every day, although patients with more severe deficiencies may require multiple checks within the day. Patients may be anemic due to folate and/or vitamin B12 deficiencies secondary to inadequate nutritional intake and require administration with one or both supplements. Decreased nutritional intake also leads to thiamine deficiencies. Although the acuity of mild folate deficiency is modest, thiamine deficiency can lead to Wernicke encephalopathy. Wernicke encephalopathy is a neurological disorder caused by thiamine deficiency [5, 14]. It can lead to various neurological symptoms and is usually associated with chronic alcoholism [5, 14]. In most alcoholic patients, oral absorption of thiamine is erratic. Initially, parenteral administration of thiamine 500 mg every hour is recommended [14]. A standard multivitamin and folate of 1 mg is also usually administered concurrently in a liter of normal saline daily for ~3 days.

Complications related to AWS also affect other areas of critical care management. Patients may have or develop gastritis, gastrointestinal bleeding, or pancreatitis that could decrease the absorption of oral medications. The management of pancreatitis generally would prevent the acute use of oral therapy [15]. AWS-related organ dysfunctions, such as liver dysfunction or cardiomyopathy, influence drug selection and dosing. Finally, because alcoholics are at greater risk for aspiration, elevation of the head of the bed to prevent aspiration and pneumonia is recommended.

Management of Alcohol Withdrawal Syndrome

Benzodiazepines

Benzodiazepines first gained their recognition for the treatment of alcohol withdrawal in a landmark study where chlordiazepoxide was determined to be the most efficacious in preventing seizures against three other drugs: chlorpromazine, hydroxyzine, and thiamine [21]. Since then, benzodiazepines have traditionally been the mainstay of treatment for alcohol withdrawal syndrome [22]. Benzodiazepines exert their effects by enhancing GABA receptor function, promoting the receptor to stay open, and allowing the influx of chloride ions into the neuron. This inhibitory effect reduces the severity of withdrawal, preventing delirium and seizures. They are effective, cheap, and conveniently can be dosed according to a fixed schedule, where the benzodiazepine is given at specific times throughout the day and additional as needed doses are available, or a symptom-triggered schedule, where the benzodiazepine is given according to the results of alcohol withdrawal scales performed. There is limited literature on whether a fixed or symptom-triggered dosing schedule is preferable for treating patients with alcohol withdrawal syndrome in an intensive care unit [23]. As benzodiazepines have exhibited treatment success for this disease state, they do not come without risks. Benzodiazepines have the potential for addiction, and dependence can result from their use. High-dose benzodiazepine therapy can lead to oversedation, respiratory depression, and even delirium [24].

There are many different medications in the class of benzodiazepines that can be utilized for alcohol withdrawal syndrome. The first benzodiazepine discovered, chlordiazepoxide, continues to be a popular choice for treating alcohol withdrawal syndrome due to its long half-life of up to 48 hours, along with diazepam, another long-acting benzodiazepine. Shorter-acting benzodiazepines such as lorazepam, oxazepam, and midazolam have also been used to manage alcohol withdrawal syndrome; however, the longer-acting benzodiazepines may provide a smoother withdrawal with their self-tapering effect. Despite that observation, there is insufficient data to prove that one benzodiazepine is superior to the other [25, 14]. Other attributes can then aid in determining which benzodiazepine to choose for specific patients, such as liver function, as well as half-life, onset of action, and cost of the drug [26]. In a 2022 meta-analysis on the different pharmacotherapies used in treating alcohol withdrawal syndrome, fixed-schedule lorazepam, diazepam, and chlordiazepoxide were superior to placebo at reducing seizure complications from alcohol withdrawal. Fixed-schedule diazepam was shown to reduce the incidence of delirium tremens, and fixed-schedule oxazepam improved endpoint CIWA scores over placebo [27].

The optimal dosing protocol for benzodiazepines to treat alcohol withdrawal syndrome in an intensive care unit has not yet been established. In a retrospective observational study conducted in the intensive care unit, intermittent lorazepam injections versus the institutional standard of continuous infusion midazolam resulted in decreased time to symptom control, a decreased amount of sedative agent required, and decreased time spent using a benzodiazepine [25]. When comparing fixed versus symptom-triggered dosing strategies in an intensive care unit, a before-and-after study showed that a symptom-triggered benzodiazepine dosing strategy was shown to result in a reduced duration of alcohol withdrawal symptoms, need for mechanical ventilation, and ICU and hospital length of stay [23]. In a non-randomized controlled trial, symptom-triggered benzodiazepine dosing also reduced alcohol-dependence relapse and cost [28].

Benzodiazepines still prove to be an efficacious treatment for alcohol withdrawal syndrome in critically ill patients. There are many options that providers can utilize while taking patient-specific characteristics into account due to the number of medications in the class as well as the different regimens that have been proven to be successful for inpatient treatment. However, reports of benzodiazepine-refractory alcohol withdrawal syndrome continue to arise, warranting the need for other treatment options for alcohol withdrawal syndrome to be studied.

Phenobarbital

Phenobarbital, a medication in the class of barbiturates, is gaining interest in patients with severe AWS that is refractory to first-line benzodiazepine treatment [29].As there is limited literature on the dose of benzodiazepine that determines refractory-AWS, or benzodiazepine failure, a cohort of 19 patients points to an excess of 50 mg of diazepam or 10 mg of lorazepam in the first hour, or an excess of 200 mg diazepam or 40 mg of lorazepam within four hours of treatment initiation, as possible thresholds [30]. Another retrospective cohort study of 54 patients considered refractory AWS to be an excess of 40 mg of diazepam needed in one hour, up to 150 mg per dose [31]. Phenobarbital acts on GABA receptors, binding to an allosteric site that allows for inhibition of the receptor without the presence of the GABA neurotransmitter. This increases the duration that the GABA chloride channel is opened for. Along with phenobarbital's long half-life and additional inhibitory effect on glutamate receptors, it can offer advantages over traditional benzodiazepine therapy, especially with the increasing need to escalate doses [32]. However, it is important to note that phenobarbital should not be used in patients with hepatic encephalopathy, liver failure, or concomitant drugs that are metabolized by cytochrome P450 3A4.

Phenobarbital presents itself as an attractive choice for monotherapy in treating AWS. It produces no active metabolites and has a half-life of a mean average of 80 hours, eliminating the need to slowly taper the regimen [33]. As serum levels can be measured, therapy with phenobarbital can be tightly controlled and adjusted as needed. Phenobarbital can be given intravenously, intramuscularly, or orally, and its low cost attributes to its popularity in treating AWS. In a retrospective observational study of 81 patients with severe AWS, determined by pre-ICU CIWA-Ar scores >15, phenobarbital was initiated when the patient was admitted to the medial ICU. In all patient encounters, phenobarbital had successful control of the patient's AWS based on a RASS score of 0 to −1, allowing transfer to the general medical floor for continued care. The primary endpoint, respiratory distress specifically from the phenobarbital use, was not seen, as no patient underwent intubation due to the sole use of phenobarbital, supported by the similar phenobarbital doses used in both intubated and non-intubated patients [33]. Another retrospective cohort study of 120 patients also found that when AWS was treated with a phenobarbital protocol, compared to a standard benzodiazepine symptom-triggered protocol, patients had significantly shorter stays in the ICU and hospital, along with lower rates of mechanical ventilation and use of adjunctive agents for symptom control [34]. A prospective placebo-controlled double-blind trial found that patients who received phenobarbital with benzodiazepines had fewer ICU admissions [35]. A 2023 meta-analysis for the use of phenobarbital in AWS concludes that this drug can be an effective tool in an ICU setting; however, the need for uniformity in dosing and further clinical trials is warranted for its consideration of use [36].

Previous studies have used a phenobarbital loading dose of 10 mg/kg followed by additional doses every 30 minutes ranging from 60 to 260 mg [34, 35, 20]. In a retrospective before-after study comparing front-loaded phenobarbital (10 mg/kg actual body weight) to low-intermittent phenobarbital (260 mg × 1, followed by 130 mg every 15 minutes as needed) for benzodiazepine-resistant AWS in a medical ICU, the front-loaded dosing strategy resulted in less mechanically ventilated patients than the low-intermittent dosing strategy [37]. It is important to mention that the study incorporated phenobarbital as an adjunct to lorazepam rather than using it as monotherapy. Additionally, the front-loaded dosing approach could be augmented with further phenobarbital doses at the discretion of the clinician. In a retrospective, quasi-experimental study, an average dose of phenobarbital (9 mg/kg ideal body weight) was used, where the researchers found an increase in hospital and ICU length of stay, which could have been skewed by the phenobarbital group patients having a significantly higher severity of alcohol withdrawal syndrome based on APACHE II scores [4]. In general, phenobarbital shows great potential as a treatment for alcohol withdrawal syndrome. It may have a safer profile than benzodiazepines, leading to shorter stays in the ICU and hospital, as well as a reduced need for intubation. However, there is currently limited evidence available, and multicenter randomized controlled trials with a proper dosing protocol are needed [38].

Propofol

Propofol is a powerful sedative-hypnotic agent that is familiar to ICU practitioners. It is a versatile sedative that is commonly used for surgical anesthesia as well as the sedation of mechanically ventilated ICU patients. Propofol is a direct agonist of $GABA_A$ receptors, binding to a site on the β-subunit of the postsynaptic $GABA_A$

receptor that is separate from the benzodiazepine subunit [39]. It also exerts an inhibitory effect on the NMDA receptor, reducing the excitatory activity of glutamate [40]. Propofol exhibits a desirable pharmacokinetic profile with a rapid onset and relatively short context-sensitive half-life, facilitating easy titration to achieve clinical targets [39].

Due to its mechanism of action as well as its anticonvulsant properties, propofol can play an important synergistic role as an adjunctive therapy in the treatment of alcohol withdrawal syndrome [40]. Because propofol can cause profound respiratory depression, mechanical ventilation is generally required, making it a reasonable option in patients that are already intubated [40]. Several retrospective studies and case reports have attempted to define the optimal role of propofol for AWS; however, the generalizability of these studies is limited by their use of various dosing strategies, the severity of symptoms, and definitions of refractory AWS. Propofol is reported to demonstrate a reduced cross-tolerance to alcohol compared to BZDs and, therefore, may offer an advantage to benzodiazepines dose-escalation in refractory AWS and delirium tremens [40]. However, two retrospective studies that compared benzodiazepines monotherapy with the addition of propofol in mechanically ventilated patients with refractory AWS demonstrated a decrease in benzodiazepines administration but similar or even worse clinical outcomes with the addition of propofol [41, 42]. Because these are retrospective studies with small sample sizes, it is possible that the patients receiving propofol were experiencing more severe symptoms, which could have confounded the results.

Propofol has also been compared to dexmedetomidine as an adjunctive agent (Table 2.2). In general, studies demonstrate that patients that receive propofol for severe AWS experience longer intubation times and ICU lengths of stay compared to those who receive dexmedetomidine [43–45]. Based on the currently available literature, the use of propofol should generally be limited to mechanically intubated patients for whom other agents have failed or are not clinically appropriate [43]. It should also be noted that in addition to respiratory depression, other risks of propofol include dose-limiting hypotension, and although rare, prolonged infusions of high doses can result in Propofol Related Infusion Syndrome (PRIS), which can be life-threatening [40].

Ketamine

Although ketamine has been available for many years, its use for sedation and analgesia in the ICU has surged in the last decade. Ketamine is a non-competitive antagonist of NMDA receptors that achieves dose-dependent dissociative sedation and theoretically should be efficacious as an adjunctive agent in refractory AWS [46, 47]. However, only recently has evidence emerged that evaluates ketamine in this population. Ketamine may even play a role in the modulation of alcohol use disorder to reduce cravings and improve abstinence [47]. Currently, two small studies demonstrate that the use of ketamine as an adjunctive agent can reduce

Table 2.2 Adjunct agents

Agent	Mechanism of action	Dose range	Clinical pearls
Baclofen	$GABA_B$ receptor agonist	50–150 mg per day	Less sedating than benzodiazepines and barbiturates Provides an alternate mechanism of GABA receptor activation Monitor for renal impairment Lack of intravenous formulation
Gabapentin	GABA neurotransmission by blocking the α2δ subunit of voltage-dependent calcium channels	900–1800 mg/day	Less sedating than benzodiazepines and barbiturates Safer side effect profile Lack of intravenous formulation
Ketamine	Antagonizes NMDA	0.15–0.3 mg/kg/hour	Rapid onset of action and short half-life Devoid of respiratory depression, does not require mechanical ventilation Targets GABA and NMDA receptor *Caution*: Delirium and hallucination may occur
Propofol	$GABA_A$-agonist and antagonizes NMDA receptors	5–60 mcg/kg/minute	Rapid onset of action; short half-life if not used for prolonged time Familiarity with ICU providers with dosing and titration *Caution*: The patient needs to be on a ventilator due to respiratory depression, hypotension, bradycardia, and propofol infusion syndrome
Dexmedetomidine	Selective a2-agonist	0.4–1.2 mcg/kg/hour	Rapid onset and offset action; less sedating than benzodiazepines, barbiturates, and propofol; lack of respiratory depression *Caution*: Cardiovascular-related side effects (↓HR ↓BP); lacks anti-seizure activity
Phenobarbital	GABA-agonist and antagonizes NMDA receptors	Front load: 10 mg/kg Bolus dosing: maximum 25 mg/kg per day	Drug-drug interactions; avoid in patients with cirrhosis; monitor for hypotension and respiratory depression Long half-life allows for auto-taper

benzodiazepine doses. The dosing in these studies ranged from sub-dissociative dosing (0.21 mg/kg/hour) to dissociative dosing (0.76 mg/kg/hour) [47]. Another study evaluating 63 patients with AWS demonstrated that the implementation of a ketamine protocol resulted in reduced intubation rates (76% vs. 29%) and ICU LOS (11.2 days vs. 5.7 days) [47]. In this study, the average dose was 0.15–0.3 mg/kg/hour [47]

Although these studies are very promising, the optimal use, timing, and dose of ketamine in AWS, especially compared to other adjunctive agents, is yet to be elucidated. An attractive feature of ketamine is that it offers a unique hemodynamic profile by stimulating the sympathetic nervous system to produce tachycardia and hypertension with minimal respiratory depression [46]. It can lead to hypersalivation and an emergence phenomenon, which includes vivid dreams and hallucinations that typically occur at higher doses [46].

Dexmedetomidine/Clonidine

Centrally acting α_2-adrenergic receptor agonists, such as dexmedetomidine (DEX) and clonidine, have been utilized in AWS treatment. Its inhibition of norepinephrine release at the locus coeruleus reduces the sympathetic effects that patients commonly present with during AWS and provides anxiolytic and sedative effects [48]. Because DEX has a relatively fast onset of action, can be administered as a continuous intravenous infusion regardless of patients' intubation status, and is easily titratable, it has become a desirable option for providers who are looking to control patients' withdrawal symptoms quickly [48]. However, it is important to note that these agents exert no activity on GABA receptor sites and therefore do not prevent withdrawal-related seizures. DEX and clonidine should not be used as monotherapy for the treatment of AWS [48]. The American Society of Addiction Medicine (ASAM) recommends that both agents can be utilized as an adjunct to benzodiazepines to control alcohol withdrawal symptoms, such as autonomic hyperactivity and anxiety, if not controlled by benzodiazepines alone; specifically for DEX, the ASAM guidelines also recommend it may be used in patients who experience resistant alcohol withdrawal symptoms in the ICU [2, 49].

Evidence for the use of clonidine in AWS is scarce, with only two randomized controlled trials published that each utilize different dosing strategies and preparations (transdermal patch and oral tablets) and have conflicting results when studied against benzodiazepines [3, 4, 50, 51]. Evidence for the use of DEX has primarily been retrospective in nature, along with two single-center, randomized controlled trials that were published. When utilized adjunctively to benzodiazepines, both trials showed DEX reduced 24-hour benzodiazepine requirements and agitation scores, but patients in the DEX group also experienced an increased incidence of bradycardia and hypotension [5, 6, 52, 53]. The use of other adjunctive medications such as phenobarbital and haloperidol was allowed in these studies, which could have limited or skewed these results. A recent meta-analysis, which included both cohort and randomized studies assessing adjunct DEX use to benzodiazepines, showed conflicting outcomes in terms of ICU length of stay, hospital length of stay, and total benzodiazepines requirements [7, 54]. The authors recognize the low quality of evidence available to establish concrete conclusions regarding the efficacy of DEX therapy and emphasize the need for more prospective, randomized controlled trials to be performed.

While DEX is primarily utilized as an adjunctive treatment to benzodiazepines, continual assessment for the appropriateness of therapy is needed as DEX may often mask patients' symptoms of withdrawal and delay appropriate administration of benzodiazepines or other therapies that may prevent alcohol-related seizures or delirium. Other considerations when discussing the continuation of therapy include the need for ICU admission when receiving DEX, which can contribute to an unnecessary and prolonged ICU length of stay as well as additional incurred medical costs. Further studies are needed to identify the subgroup of patients who may benefit from DEX therapy the most, such as those with resistant or refractory withdrawal, and how to best incorporate this therapy into AWS protocols.

Gabapentin

Recently, several studies have attempted to characterize the potential role of gabapentin, an anxiolytic and anticonvulsant drug with analgesic properties, as a benzodiazepine-sparing treatment modality for AWS in outpatient and inpatient settings [55]. Gabapentin inhibits voltage-gated calcium channels and indirectly increases the activity of endogenous GABA concentrations without directly stimulating GABA receptors [55, 56]. Although the evidence is limited and inconsistent, available studies demonstrate that gabapentin, either alone or in combination with other agents, may be efficacious in reducing insomnia and cravings in patients with alcohol dependence, which can help prevent relapse in the early abstinence phase [55]. In a randomized trial of 90 patients with self-reported alcohol withdrawal symptoms who abstained from alcohol for at least three days, a 16-week regimen of gabapentin escalated to a dose of 1200 mg/day was found to reduce heavy drinking days and increase total abstinence [56].

A meta-analysis of eight retrospective studies of gabapentin in hospitalized patients with AWS demonstrated that gabapentin, either alone or in combination with benzodiazepines, was associated with some improvements in outcomes, including reduced length of stay and benzodiazepine doses, but the studies were at high risk of bias and confounding [57].The doses of gabapentin used in these studies varied greatly, but doses greater than 1800 mg/day appear to be the most effective [57]. Although it is plausible that gabapentin can serve as a valuable adjunct in severe AWS and possibly monotherapy in mild withdrawal, the authors concluded that more studies are needed before gabapentin can be recommended routinely for AWS [57]. This is especially true for severe withdrawal requiring intensive care, patients at high risk of delirium tremens or seizures, or patients with complicated medical or psychiatric comorbidities [55]. This agent may be especially useful in patients who are willing to continue gabapentin beyond the acute phase of alcohol withdrawal as a strategy to prevent relapses, especially when benzodiazepines are discontinued [55, 58].

Clinicians should be aware that gabapentin doses require adjustment in renal failure, and abrupt discontinuation of gabapentin can also result in a withdrawal syndrome, which may result in symptoms that mirror AWS [55]. Finally, although side effects are typically minimal, an important potential concern of gabapentin is the potential for abuse, which has been described recently but is likely to be less relevant than with benzodiazepines [58, 59].

Baclofen

Baclofen is FDA-approved for the treatment of muscle spasticity, but it has also been used off-label for the treatment of alcohol withdrawal syndrome (AWS). Baclofen's exact mechanism of action in AWS remains unclear, but it is thought that its activation on $GABA_B$ receptors impairs dopaminergic release in the brain, resulting in reduced cravings and consumption of alcohol [60]. The most common dosing strategy utilized for this indication is 30 mg per day in three divided doses, but regimens remain varied in clinical practice. Given the limited and very low quality of evidence from two meta-analyses comparing the efficacy and safety of baclofen against either placebo or benzodiazepines, baclofen should not be considered a first-line agent for AWS treatment but rather as an adjunct or a benzodiazepine-sparing regimen [61, 62]. However, a recent randomized controlled trial by Vourc'h and colleagues has assessed its utility in the prevention of agitation due to alcohol withdrawal [4, 63]. This was the first study that assessed baclofen use against placebo for the prevention of agitation-related events in patients at high risk of alcohol withdrawal on mechanical ventilation for at least 24 hours. Patients in the baclofen group received a loading dose between 50 and 150 mg based on their estimated glomerular filtration rate (eGFR) on day 1 and then doses of 50–150 mg in three divided doses up until day 15. Doses were tapered and discontinued upon discharge from the intensive care unit (ICU). For the primary outcome, there was a statistically significant reduction in the percentage of patients experiencing at least one agitation-related event in the baclofen group when compared to the placebo group (19.7% versus 29.7%, respectively; $p = 0.04$). While there was no difference in mortality between the two groups ($p = 0.44$), patients receiving baclofen, when compared to placebo, did have longer lengths of mechanical ventilation (9 days versus 8 days, $p = 0.02$), ICU stay (14 days versus 11 days, $p = 0.01$), and delayed awakening requiring drug discontinuation (8.9% versus 1.9%), which highlights baclofen's sedative effects. Further studies are needed to determine the optimal dosing strategy of baclofen as well as its role in preventing alcohol withdrawal-induced agitation.

Clinical Implications and Conclusions

AWS is a common condition encountered in the ICU that requires careful attention due to the high risk of severe complications. Managing AWS in the ICU requires a multidisciplinary approach. Validated assessment tools, such as the CIWA-Ar, RASS, or SAS scales, can help assess symptom severity and guide treatment decisions. Pharmacological interventions, primarily benzodiazepines, phenobarbital, and various adjuncts, are commonly used to manage AWS symptoms and prevent complications. It is crucial to closely monitor vital signs, neurological status, and organ function to identify and manage complications such as seizures, delirium, cardiovascular instability, and metabolic disturbances. Although there are numerous agents available for managing AWS, larger multicenter prospective randomized controlled trials are necessary to determine optimal treatment options.

References

1. Moore RD, Bone LR, Geller G, Mamon JA, Stokes EJ, Levine DM. Prevalence, detection, and treatment of alcoholism in hospitalized patients. JAMA. 1989;261(3):403–7. PMID: 2909780.
2. National Survey on Drug Use and Health. Available from www.samhsa.gov/data. Accessed 15 June 2023.
3. Awissi DK, Lebrun G, Fagnan M, et al. Alcohol, nicotine, and iatrogenic withdrawals in the ICU. Crit Care Med. 2013;41:S57–68.
4. Ferreira JA, Wieruszewski PM, Cunningham DW, Davidson KE, Weisberg SF. Approach to the complicated alcohol withdrawal patient. J Intensive Care Med. 2017;32(1):3–14. https://doi.org/10.1177/0885066615614273. Epub 2015 Oct 30. PMID: 26518697.
5. Carlson RW, Kumar NN, Wong-Mckinstry E, et al. Alcohol withdrawal syndrome. Crit Care Clin. 2012;28:549–85.
6. Jesse S, Bråthen G, Ferrara M, et al. Alcohol withdrawal syndrome: mechanisms, manifestations, and management. ActaNeurol Scand. 2017;135:4–16.
7. Saitz R, O'Malley SS. Pharmacotherapies for alcohol abuse. Withdrawal and treatment. Med Clin North Am. 1997;81:881–907.
8. DeBellis R, Smith BS, Choi S, et al. Management of delirium tremens. J Intensive Care Med. 2005;20:164–73.
9. Marik P, Mohedin B. Alcohol-related admissions to an inner city hospital intensive care unit. Alcohol Alcoholism. 1996;31:393–6.
10. Sacks JJ, Gonzales KR, Bouchery EE, et al. 2010 national and state costs of excessive alcohol consumption. Am J Prev Med. 2015;49:e73–9.
11. Saitz R. Introduction to alcohol withdrawal. Alcohol Health Res World. 1998;22:5–12.
12. American Psychiatric Association. Diagnostic and statistical manual of mental disorders, DSM-5. 5th ed. Washington, DC: American Psychiatric Publishing; 2013.
13. Clark BJ, Keniston A, Douglas IS, et al. Healthcare utilization in medical intensive care unit survivors with alcohol withdrawal. Alcohol Clin Exp Res. 2013;37:1536–43.
14. Perry EC. Inpatient management of acute alcohol withdrawal syndrome. CNS Drugs. 2014;28:401–10.
15. McKeon A, Frye MA, Delanty N. The alcohol withdrawal syndrome. J Neurol Neurosurg Psychiatry. 2008;79:854–62.
16. Mayo-Smith MF. Pharmacologic management of alcohol withdrawal: a meta-analysis and evidence-based practice guideline. JAMA. 1997;278(2):144–51.

17. Saitz R, Mayo-Smith MF, Roberts MS, Redmond HA, Bernard DR, Calkins DR. Individualized treatment for alcohol withdrawal. A randomized double-blind controlled trial. JAMA. 1994;272(7):519–23.
18. Daeppen JB, Gache P, Landry U, et al. Symptom-triggered vs fixed-scheduled doses of benzodiazepines for alcohol withdrawal: a randomized treatment trial. Arch Intern Med. 2002;162(10):1117–21.
19. Sullivan JT, Sykora K, Schneiderman J, Naranjo CA, Sellers EM. Assessment of alcohol withdrawal: the revised clinical institute withdrawal assessment for alcohol scale (CIWA-Ar). Br J Addict. 1989;84(11):1353–7.
20. Duby JJ, Berry AJ, Ghayyem P, Wilson MD, Cocanour CS. Alcohol withdrawal syndrome in critically ill patients: protocolized versus nonprotocolized management. J Trauma Acute Care Surg. 2014;77:938–43.
21. Kaim SC, Klett CJ, Rothfeld B. Treatment of the acute alcohol withdrawal state: a comparison of four drugs. Am J Psychiatry. 1969;125:1640–6.
22. Spies C, Dubisz N, Neumann T, Blum S, Muller C, Rommelspacher H, Brummer G, Specht M, Sanft C, Hannemann L, Striebel H, Schaffartzik W. Therapy of alcohol withdrawal syndrome in intensive care unit patients following trauma. Crit Care Med. 1996;24(3):414–22.
23. Sen S, Grgurich P, Tulolo A, Smith-Freedman A, Lei Y, Gray A, Dargin J. A symptom-triggered benzodiazepine protocol utilizing SAS and CIWA-Ar scoring for the treatment of alcohol withdrawal syndrome in the critically ill. Ann Pharmacother. 2017;51(2):101–10.
24. DeCarolis DD, Rice KL, Ho L, et al. Symptom-driven lorazepam protocol for treatment of severe alcohol withdrawal delirium in the intensive care unit. Pharmacotherapy. 2007;27:510–8.
25. Weintraub SJ. Diazepam in the treatment of moderate to severe alcohol withdrawal. CNS Drugs. 2017;31(2):87–95.
26. Sarff M, Gold JA. Alcohol withdrawal syndromes in the intensive care unit. Crit Care Med. 2010;38(9 Suppl):S494–501.
27. Bahji A, Bach P, Danilewitz M, Crockford D, El-Guebaly N, Devoe DJ, Saitz R. Comparative efficacy and safety of pharmacotherapies for alcohol withdrawal: a systematic review and network meta-analysis. Addiction. 2022;117(10):2591–601.
28. Al-Maqbali JS, Al Alawi AM, Al-Mamari Q, Al-Huraizi A, Al-Maqrashi N. Symptoms-triggered approach versus fixed-scheduled approach of benzodiazepines for management of alcohol withdrawal syndrome: non-randomized controlled trial. Alcohol. 2023 Feb;106:10–4.
29. Umar Z, Haseeb Ul Rasool M, Muhammad S, et al. Phenobarbital and alcohol withdrawal syndrome: a systematic review and meta-analysis. Cureus. 2023;15(1):e33695.
30. Hack JB, Hoffman RS, Nelson LS. Resistant alcohol withdrawal: does an unexpectedly large sedative requirement identify these patients early? J Med Toxic. 2006;2(2):55–60.
31. Gold JA, Rimal B, Nolan A, Nelson LS. A strategy of escalating doses of benzodiazepines and phenobarbital administration reduces the need for mechanical ventilation in delirium tremens. Crit Care Med. 2007 Mar;35(3):724–30.
32. Goodberlet M, Dube K, Kovacevic M, Szumita P, DeGrado J. Evaluation of a phenobarbital-based protocol for severe alcohol withdrawal in critically ill patients. Hosp Pharm. 2021;56(5):550–9.
33. Oks M, Cleven KL, Healy L, Wei M, Narasimhan M, Mayo PH, Kohn N, Koenig S. The safety and utility of phenobarbital use for the treatment of severe alcohol withdrawal syndrome in the medical intensive care unit. J Intensive Care Med. 2020;35(9):844–50.
34. Tidwell WP, Thomas TL, Pouliot JD, Canonico AE, Webber AJ. Treatment of alcohol withdrawal syndrome: phenobarbital vs CIWA-Ar protocol. Am J Crit Care. 2018;27:454–60.
35. Rosenson J, Clements C, Simon B, Vieaux J, Graffman S, Vahidnia F, Cisse B, Lam J, Alter H. Phenobarbital for acute alcohol withdrawal: a prospective randomized double-blind placebo-controlled study. J Emerg Med. 2013;44(3):592–598.e2.
36. Umar Z, Haseeb Ul Rasool M, Muhammad S, Yousaf S, Nassar M, Ilyas U, Hosna AU, Parikh A, Bhangal R, Ahmed N, Ariyaratnam J, Trandafirescu T. Phenobarbital and alcohol withdrawal syndrome: a systematic review and meta-analysis. Cureus. 2023;15(1):e33695.

37. Shah P, Stegner-Smith KL, Rachid M, Hanif T, Dodd KW. Front-loaded versus low-intermittent phenobarbital dosing for benzodiazepine-resistant severe alcohol withdrawal syndrome. J Med Toxicol. 2022;18(3):198–204.
38. Nishimura Y, Choi H, Colgan B, Kistler H, Mercado F. Current evidence and clinical utility of phenobarbital for alcohol withdrawal syndrome. Eur J Intern Med. 2023;17:S0953-6205(23)00084-5.
39. Sahinovic MM, Struys MMRF, Absalom AR. Clinical pharmacokinetics and pharmacodynamics of propofol. Clin Pharmacokinet. 2018;57:1539–58.
40. Brotherton AL, Hamilton EP, Kloss HG, et al. Propofol for the treatment of refractory alcohol withdrawal syndrome: a review of the literature. Pharmacotherapy. 2016;36(4):433–42. https://doi.org/10.1002/phar.1726.
41. Wong A, Benedict NJ, Lohr BR, et al. Management of benzodiazepine-resistant alcohol withdrawal across a healthcare system: benzodiazepine dose-escalation with or without propofol. Drug Alcohol Depend. 2015;154:296–9.
42. Sohraby R, Attridge RL, Hughes DW. Use of propofol-containing versus benzodiazepine regimens for alcohol withdrawal requiring mechanical ventilation. Ann Pharmacother. 2014;48(4):456–61. https://doi.org/10.1177/1060028013515846.
43. Ludtke KA, Stanley KS, Yount NL, et al. Retrospective review of critically ill patients experiencing alcohol withdrawal: dexmedetomidine versus propofol and/or lorazepam continuous infusions. Hosp Pharm. 2015;50(3):208–13.
44. Lizotte RJ, Kappes JA, Bartel BJ, et al. Evaluating the effects of dexmedetomidine compared to propofol as adjunctive therapy in patients with alcohol withdrawal. Clin Pharmacol Adv Appl. 2014;6:171–7.
45. Love K, Zimmermann AE. Use of propofol plus Dexmedetomidine in patients experiencing severe alcohol withdrawal in the intensive care unit. J Clin Pharmacol. 2020;60(4):439–43.
46. Midega TD, Chaves RCF, Ashihara C, et al. Ketamine use in critically ill patients: a narrative review. Rev Bras Ter Intensiva. 2022;34(2):287–94. https://doi.org/10.5935/0103-507X.20220027-pt.
47. Goldfine CE, Tom JJ, Im DD, et al. The therapeutic use and efficacy of ketamine in alcohol use disorder and alcohol withdrawal syndrome: a scoping review. Front Psych. 2023;14:1141836. https://doi.org/10.3389/fpsyt.2023.1141836.
48. Gertler R, Brown HC, Mitchell DH, Silvius EN. Dexmedetomidine: a novel sedative-analgesic agent. Proc (Bayl Univ Med Cent). 2001;14(1):13–21.
49. Alvanzo A, Kleinschmidt K, Kmiec JA, et al. The ASAM clinical practice guideline on alcohol withdrawal management. J Addict Med. 2020;14(3S Suppl 1):1–72.
50. Adinoff B. Double-blind study of alprazolam, diazepam, clonidine, and placebo in the alcohol withdrawal syndrome: preliminary findings. Alcohol Clin Exp Res. 1994;18(4):873–8.
51. Baumgartner GR, Rowen RC. Transdermal clonidine versus chlordiazepoxide in alcohol withdrawal: a randomized, controlled clinical trial. South Med J. 1991;84(3):312–21.
52. Muller SW, Preslaski CR, Kiser TH, et al. A randomized, double-blind, placebo-controlled dose range study of dexmedetomidine as adjunctive therapy for alcohol withdrawal. Crit Care Med. 2014;42(5):1131–9.
53. Bielka K, Kuchyn I, Glumcher F. Addition of dexmedetomidine to benzodiazepines for patients with alcohol withdrawal syndrome in the intensive care unit: a randomized controlled study. Ann Intensive Care. 2015;5(1):33.
54. Polintan ETT, Danganan LML, Crus NS, et al. Adjunctive dexmedetomidine in alcohol withdrawal syndrome: a systematic review and meta-analysis of retrospective cohort studies and randomized controlled trials. Ann Pharmacother. 2023;57(6):696–705.
55. Leung JG, Hall-Flavin D, Nelson S, et al. The role of gabapentin in the management of alcohol withdrawal and dependence. Ann Pharmacother. 2015;49(8):897–906. https://doi.org/10.1177/1060028015585849.
56. Anton RF, Latham P, Voronin K, et al. Efficacy of gabapentin for the treatment of alcohol use disorder in patients with alcohol withdrawal symptoms: a randomized clinical trial. JAMA Intern Med. 2020;180(5):728–36. https://doi.org/10.1001/jamainternmed.2020.0249.

57. Mattle AG, McGrath P, Sanu A, et al. Gabapentin to treat acute alcohol withdrawal in hospitalized patients: a systematic review and meta-analysis. Drug Alcohol Depend. 2022;241:109671. https://doi.org/10.1016/j.drugalcdep.2022.109671.
58. Bates RE, Leung JG, Morgan RJ, et al. Retrospective analysis of gabapentin for alcohol withdrawal in the hospital setting: the mayo clinic experience. Mayo Clin Proc Inn Qual Out. 2020;4(5):542–9.
59. Modesto-Lowe V, Barron GC, Aronow B, et al. Gabapentin for alcohol use disorder: a good option, or cause for concern? Cleveland Clinic Journal of Medicine. 2019;86(12):815–23. https://doi.org/10.3949/ccjm.86a.18128.
60. de Beaurepaire R. A review of the potential mechanisms of action of baclofen in alcohol use disorder. Front Psych. 2018;9:506.
61. Liu J, Wang LN. Baclofen for alcohol withdrawal. Cochrane Database Syst Rev. 2019;11:CD008502.
62. Ghosh A, Mahintamani T, Choudhury S, Sharma N, Das S. The effectiveness of non-benzodiazepine, non-barbiturate medications for alcohol withdrawal syndrome: a rapid systematic review. Alcohol Alcohol. 2021;56(5):513–34.
63. Vourc'h M, Garret C, Gacouin A, et al. Effect of high-dose baclofen on agitation-related events among patients with unhealthy alcohol use receiving mechanical ventilation: a randomized clinical trial. JAMA. 2021;325(8):732–41.

Chapter 3
Alcohol Use Disorder and Critical Illness

Akhil Patel

Abbreviations

ARDS	Acute respiratory distress syndrome
AUD	Alcohol use disorder
GABA	Gamma-aminobutyric acid
ICU	Intensive care unit
NMDA	N-methyl-d-aspartate
OSA	Obstructive sleep apnea
RSV	Respiratory syncytial disease
SVR	Systemic vascular resistance

Introduction

Alcohol use disorder (AUD) is the inability of patients to control alcohol consumption even in the setting of adverse medical, psychological, social, and financial consequences [1]. Diagnostic criteria for AUD have been changed to now incorporate both the diagnoses of alcohol abuse and dependence, as well as create a spectrum of severity. Eleven criteria encompass a questionnaire to assess the level of disorder, with mild disease having 2–3 affirmations, moderate disease having 4–5 positive answers, and severe disease defined as 6 or more positive answers [1, 2] (Table 3.1). Based on the 2021 National Survey on Drug Use and Health, over 28 million adults over the age of 18 were diagnosed with AUD [1]. In 2020, over 250,000 hospital admissions were due to alcohol use alone, with another 200,000 admissions with

A. Patel (✉)
Department of Anesthesiology and Critical Care Medicine, George Washington University School of Medicine and Health Sciences, Washington, DC, USA

K. Karamchandani, J. E. Grant (eds.), *Substance Use Disorders in Adult Critically Ill Patients*, https://doi.org/10.1007/978-3-031-67069-5_3

Table 3.1 Alcohol use disorder 11 criteria questionnaire

Alcohol use disorder DSM 5 questionnaire	
1	Do you drink more than you plan on?
2	Have you failed at cutting down on or stopping consumption more than once?
3	Do you spend most of your time drinking or recovering from the side effects?
4	Have you had difficulties concentrating because of an urge to drink?
5	Has drinking interfered with family, work, or school?
6	Do you continue to drink in spite of interference with family, work, or school?
7	Have you decreased your time with your hobbies in order to drink?
8	Have you unintentionally placed yourself in harmful situations while or due to drinking? (swimming, driving, unprotected sex)
9	Have you continued drinking despite memory loss, mental illness, or other health illnesses?
10	Have you noticed requiring more drinks to achieve the same effect?
11	Have you ever experienced withdrawal symptoms (shaking, nausea, racing heart, seizures)?

A positive response in 2–3 questions results in mild disease; 4–5 questions result in moderate disease; and more than 6 results in severe disease. The questions are asked in reference to the past year

alcohol as a secondary substance used [3]. This trend is not limited to the United States, as the overall incidence of alcohol consumption is increasing worldwide [4].

As the incidence of AUD increases, it is important to understand the systemic effects of alcohol on various organ systems to assist with the management of patients with AUD, which can be seen in image 1 below. These patients have a high propensity for complications during their hospital stay and are progressing to a critical status. Liver failure and encephalopathy are perhaps the most associated with AUD; however, each organ system is affected. Although causality is not always proven, AUD has been associated with worse outcomes. The effects of alcohol on each organ system and the pathophysiology of the development of various alcohol-related complications will be discussed.

Neurological/Psychological

Alcohol use disorder is a psychiatric disorder characterized by the inability of the patient to control consumption of alcohol despite detrimental consequences to themselves and others [5]. A majority of patients admitted to the ICU with AUD are due to alcohol withdrawal syndrome (AWS). Alcohol upregulates the neurological depressant gamma-aminobutyric acid (GABA) and simultaneously inhibits N-methyl-d-aspartate (NMDA), an excitant. The chronicity of the disorder downregulates GABA receptors and upregulates NMDA receptors. Acute cessation of alcohol consumption leads to an unbalanced excitation phase, leading to the manifestation of AWS, which can range from delirium and agitation to hemodynamic collapse and seizures [6, 7]. Delirium tremens is the most severe presentation of alcohol withdrawal, with symptoms of autonomic hyperactivity, hyperemesis, hallucinations, seizures, and delirium [8]. It is important to note that AUD increases sedation requirements. Patients require higher amounts of adjuncts and may require higher doses of typical sedation in order to achieve optimal sedation because of the aforementioned neurotransmitter imbalances along with the upregulation of dopamine, leading to further hyperexcitation [6, 7, 9, 10].

Wernicke-Korsakoff syndrome is a neurological syndrome with an initial presentation of peripheral neuropathy, gait imbalance, and encephalopathy, and patients can develop psychosis and memory loss. Wernicke's encephalopathy manifests acutely, whereas Kosakoff syndrome usually presents in a chronic fashion. AUD diminishes the ability to absorb thiamine across the intestinal wall, thus increasing the risk of Wernicke-Korsakoff syndrome. Often overlooked, thiamine is integral for various cerebellar and brainstem processes, which can be irreversibly damaged by neuronal damage [11]. It is worth mentioning that AUD is often associated with other psychiatric disorders [12, 13], and it is unclear if AUD is the cause or risk factor for the development of these disorders. Violent and aggressive behavior and other substance use heighten the risk for AUD and can further complicate the management of critically ill patients [12, 13].

Cardiovascular

AUD is a known risk factor for hypertension, high-output cardiac failure, and atrial fibrillation [6, 14]. Although the mechanism is not clear, there are many factors causing AUD-induced hypertension. The consumption of alcohol may increase sympathetic discharge, possibly due to increased cortisol levels [15]. Alcohol has also been found to stimulate endothelin 1 and 2, angiotensin II, and norepinephrine secretion, which are all potent vasoconstrictors. Elevated intracellular calcium has been noted to increase the sensitivity of norepinephrine effects on systemic vascular resistance (SVR) [15]. It is important to remember that hypertension is also a sign of AWS, thus making the differentiation difficult to make.

Heart failure related to alcohol use can present in the form of high output failure or dilated cardiomyopathy [16, 17]. Wet beriberi is a manifestation of thiamine deficiency resulting in shortness of breath, lower extremity swelling, tachycardia due to cardiac failure, right heart failure, and acidosis [16]. Thiamine deficiency leads to a decrease in adenosine triphosphate production which in turn reduces SVR and augments venous return, causing an extremely high cardiac output [16]. However, this unsustainable output eventually leads to heart failure and a low output state. Dilated cardiomyopathy may be a consequence of this high output failure, along with elevated toxic metabolites such as reactive oxygen species [17]. Autonomic hyperreactivity due to withdrawal symptoms can be extremely detrimental in these patients with compromised cardiac function and must be monitored closely.

Alcohol-mediated adrenal secretion, increased circulating levels of norepinephrine and epinephrine, oxidative stress, and toxic metabolites have all been linked to the development of atrial fibrillation [18]. Atrial fibrillation is one of the most common arrhythmias observed among AUD patients [18]. Other systemic effects of

AUD, which include obstructive sleep apnea (OSA), hypertension, and obesity, also increase the risk of atrial fibrillation [19]. There is a heightened concern that increased sympathetic activity in patients undergoing withdrawal may also precipitate atrial fibrillation.

Pulmonary

AUD has been associated with a higher percentage of intubation and mechanical ventilation in ICU patients. There is an almost 50% increase in the risk of mechanical ventilation in AUD patients, and AWS has also been linked to longer durations of mechanical ventilation [20]. The risks for ventilator-associated pneumonias are worsened with colonization of the oropharynx, gingivodental disease, and aspiration risks associated with AUD [6]. As such, AUD patients have a high likelihood of developing acute respiratory distress syndrome (ARDS) due to their predisposition for gram-negative colonization, decreased ciliary clearance, and poor immune response, leading to endothelin dysfunction [20]. Overall, it has been estimated that AUD almost doubles the risk of developing ARDS [21].

Patients with AUD are also more likely to develop OSA. Although the causality has yet to be proven, multiple studies and meta-analyses have shown that apnea and snoring increase in a dose-dependent manner with the consumption of alcohol [22–24]. Some plausible reasons include changes in the epithelial mucosa, hypoglossal and genioglossal motor nerve weakness, and fragmentation of sleep [22].

It is important to note that the act of drinking alcohol does not by itself cause pulmonary complications. Essentially, AUD magnifies the risks associated with the development of pulmonary complications due to an initial insult, be it from an infectious etiology such as pneumonia or from a traumatic injury [20, 22].

Gastrointestinal

Alcohol use is most commonly implicated with the development of liver injury, but it is not the only organ within the gastrointestinal system that is affected by chronic alcohol consumption. To begin, alcohol is introduced to the body via the oral cavity, where it can lead to salivary gland hypertrophy, gingival disease, esophageal motility issues, and esophageal mucosa degradation and bleeding [25]. Weakening of the lower esophageal sphincter results in gastro-esophageal reflex and increases the risk for aspiration. Reflex of acidic gastric contents disrupts normal esophageal mucosa, leading to Barrett's esophagus, and can result in Mallory-Weiss syndrome, or mucosal tears at the gastro-esophageal junction [21, 25].

The gastric and intestinal mucosae are injured, like the esophageal mucosa. The risk of bleeding is very high and is a common finding in critically ill patients with AUD [25]. Many ICU admissions related to AUD are in fact due to gastrointestinal bleeding [21]. Chronic alcohol intake and weakening of the gastric mucosa lead to bacterial colonization and increased risks of infection. Poor motility is noted in patients chronically ingesting beverages with a high alcohol content [25].

Mucosal damage to the intestines leads to inappropriate absorption of nutrients, increased risk of bleeding, and metabolic and bacterial toxin absorption and transfer [25]. Malnutrition is caused due to a decreased uptake of macromolecules, along with delayed motility and overall satiety from the motility issues. Vitamins such as thiamine and B12, along with folic acid, are not absorbed, leading to the complications mentioned above as well as pernicious anemia [25]. Motility issues lead to bacterial overgrowth within the intestines, and this overgrowth leads to increased production of bacterial toxin, also creating mucosal lesions. Alcohol releases toxins which damage small vessels within the villi, causing cell death, then creating lesions and increasing the permeability of bacterial toxins and cytokines, resulting in systemic organ damage, including liver failure [25].

Acute pancreatitis is one of the most common gastrointestinal illnesses requiring hospital admission [21, 25–27]. AUD is one of the most common risk factors for the development of acute pancreatitis, along with gallstone disease. The exact pathophysiology is still unclear [26], but ethanol is known to be degraded by the pancreas in both oxidative and non-oxidative pathways within the liver as well as the pancreatic acinar cells. Generation of acetaldehyde and reactive oxygen species may cause cell death and incite an inflammatory cascade leading to acute pancreatitis [26]. Due to the rapid nature of the disease, it is unclear how an acute flare occurs. A dose-dependent causal relationship between alcohol use and acute pancreatitis has been well documented [26, 27]. Smoking, race, diet, and genetics are thought to play an additional role in the development of alcohol-related pancreatitis [27].

Both end-stage liver disease and acute liver failure are some of the most dreaded complications of AUD and often require ICU admission. AUD is the number-one cause of liver failure and cirrhosis [22]. The severity of disease can be a predictor of 1-year mortality, with 10–15% mortality within 1 month of diagnosis and 20% within 1 year for mild-moderate disease, with severe disease mortality rates of 50% at 1 month and 70% at 6 months [28]. Although supportive and medical therapies such as glucocorticoids, diuretics, and N-acetylcysteine are available, the definitive therapy is liver transplantation [28].

Although the exact etiology is unclear, potential exacerbations and causes of liver failure are similar to pancreatic degradation via oxygen radicals produced by ethanol metabolism [29]. Other etiologies include gut translocation of bacteria and toxin from destruction of small intestine villi and mucosa [25, 29].

Patients with alcohol-induced acute liver failure may present with a myriad of symptoms. Jaundice with elevated bilirubin levels, ascites, and portal hypertension are common findings. As the liver function deteriorates, gluconeogenesis, lactic acid degradation, the synthesis of Vitamin K-dependent factors, and other coagulation factors are all impaired [30]. Acute encephalopathy may be in part due to alcohol withdrawal or due to hyperammonemia [31]. Upper gastroesophageal bleeds are common due to esophageal varices and the risk of Mallory-Weiss tears. Patients can have high-output cardiac failure, as mentioned above, renal failure due to renal hypoperfusion, or hepato-renal syndrome, as well as complex pulmonary diseases such as hepatopulmonary syndrome and porto-pulmonary syndrome [31].

Renal

AUD results in many electrolyte abnormalities and renal disturbances. Hyponatremia is frequently found in laboratory workups due to free water ingestion and poor free water excretion [32]. Hypokalemia is not reflective of the total body potassium, as true intracellular potassium may still be within normal limits [32]. Alkalosis is typically noted due to volume contraction from GI losses [32]. Other electrolyte abnormalities include hypocalcemia and hypomagnesemia. Vitamin D deficiency can also be noted. All these derangements can often be explained due to malabsorption and liver failure [33].

As the liver begins to fail, the renal system is usually involved. Acidosis, hyperkalemia, hyperphosphatemia, and elevated creatinine are typically noted. Dialysis may be needed, and renal transplantation may be avoided if liver failure is addressed early in the diagnosis [32].

Endocrine

As mentioned above, AUD is connected to malnutrition with various electrolyte abnormalities. However, at the core of the diagnosis, AUD is a psychological disorder. Patients with AUD are often cachectic with muscle wasting due to poor absorption; however, there have been links to anorexia and bulimia [34]. Data has proven a causal link between neurotransmitters with AUD and eating disorders, which also include being overweight or obese. This includes corticotrophin-releasing factor and melanocortins, which increase satiety, while neuropeptide Y increases hunger [34]. A meta-analysis in 2019 confirmed these findings with a positive correlation between eating disorders and alcohol use disorder [35]. While there is a link between alcohol use disorder and diabetes, it is unclear if AUD is an independent risk factor for diabetes. There is a high likelihood of diabetes with moderate to high alcohol consumption; however, the mechanism behind this association is unclear [14, 36].

Infectious Disease

The association between AUD and infections has been well documented since as early as 1775 [37]. There are specific links to an increased risk of bacterial pneumonia, tuberculosis infections, respiratory syncytial virus (RSV), ARDS, and HIV infections [37–39]. AUD causes dysfunction within the immune system, depressing pro-inflammatory markers. AUD decreases the production of cytokines TNF-alpha and interleukin-1-beta [39]. Without these cytokines, adhesion molecules and polymorphonuclear leukocytes are not upregulated in response to a foreign substance. Polymorphonuclear leukocyte recruitment, phagocytosis, and oxidative burst have all been found to be depressed due to acute alcohol intake [38, 39]. Chronic alcohol intake has shown a decrease in overall lymphocyte count, depressing the host response [38, 39]. Specifically, interference with the function of the granulocyte colony-stimulating factory by alcohol leads to a decrease in production within the bone marrow [38]. There have also been findings consistent with decreased natural killer cell activation for tumor surveillance [39].

As mentioned above, AUD is an independent risk factor for bacterial pneumoniae and the progression to ARDS [39]. A combination of the diminished esophageal tone allowing for the increased risk of aspiration, sedative properties of alcohol, and mucociliary destruction from chronic alcohol ingestion all lead to a higher risk of pneumonia [39]. The gingival damage and gastric mucosa alterations allow for the colonization of gram-negative rods and increase the risk of pneumonia and bacterial infections in general [39]. Streptococcus pneumoniae and Klebsiella pneumoniae are the most common bacterial pneumonias associated with AUD [38, 39]. Specifically in the lungs, macrophages within the alveolar space are the primary form of innate response. However, the phagocytic function along with recruitment are severely dampened from chronic alcohol consumption [36, 37].

Similarly, there has been a high propensity for viral infections in AUD, such as RSV [38]. The protective mucociliary system is degraded due to chronic alcohol intake, and coupled with the blunted host response mentioned above, AUD increases the likelihood of toxin and viral invasion and absorption [38].

Due to this diminished immune response, AUD has been connected to higher rates of tuberculosis. In impoverished and over-populated areas, the likelihood of tuberculosis transmission is higher with more resistance [36, 38]. The decreased function of macrophages, neutrophils, and natural killer cells decreases the efficacy of routine treatment failure [37, 38].

The use of alcohol has been shown to impair decision making skills. Studies have shown evidence of alcohol impacting decision-making. In regards to HIV, the likelihood of unprotected sexual interactions has been shown to be higher in those with AUD, increasing the transmissibility of the virus [38]. Further causality of the progression of HIV and AUD is difficult to prove. Although there is an immunological depression in AUD patients, there is no concrete evidence to support a change in viral count or CD4 count due to alcohol intake. There is a rising suspicion that noncompliance of medication can be seen in AUD [38].

Hematological/Oncological

Alcohol has been categorized as group 1 carcinogenic compound by the International Agency for Cancer Research [40]. AUD has been found to have causality with many different types of cancer [40]. The main physiological link is the production of acetaldehyde, a carcinogenic metabolite of ethanol [42, 43]. Other connections include folate deficiency leading to an increase in homocysteine and inhibition of folate cycle enzymes, hormonal disruptions, alterations in insulin-like growth factor concentrations, and affinity for other substances used along with alcohol such as tobacco [40].

The American College of Clinical Oncology states that alcohol is a direct cause of cancers of the oral cavity, pharynx, larynx, esophagus (squamous cell carcinoma), colorectum, hepatocellular carcinoma, and female breast cancer [41]. The duration and amount of alcohol strongly increase the risk of oropharyngeal and laryngeal cancer [41]. However unclear, there appears to be a strong suspicion for AD as a cause of gastric and pancreatic cancer [40, 41]. Cessation may decrease the risk, but the rate of regression is unclear in relation to the duration of [41].

Musculoskeletal/Trauma

The 2016 National Trauma Data Bank Report by the American College of Surgeons reported that about 12% of all trauma patients tested positive for alcohol use [42]. Positive alcohol screens have been associated with repeat trauma related admissions [6]. Patients with AUD are known to have more injuries upon admission, require ICU admission, and have a higher morbidity and mortality [43]. Acute intoxication does not increase risk; however, chronicity of disease leads to an increase in mortality [20].

AUD-related trauma can be caused by many different factors. Neurological depressant characteristics of AUD impair balance, focus, judgement, and reaction times [44]. Alcohol has been shown to decrease glucose metabolism and increase acetate metabolism in the cerebellum, hippocampus, occipital cortex, and amygdala [44]. These areas are integral for balance, focus, judgement, and memory, which, when affected, can lead to intentional or unintentional trauma [43]. Intentional trauma includes harm to oneself and others, whereas unintentional trauma includes drowning, driving-related accidents, falls, and poisonings. As the rate of AUD increases, the number of traumas, intentional or unintentional, will increase [1, 44]. Prevention can start during initial admission with brief conversations and interventions [6]. Follow-up visits and frequent brief encounters related to AUD during admissions have been found to dramatically decrease recurrent trauma related admissions [6].

Conclusion

AUD is a dynamic disease process that affects every organ system. Early intervention in patients with AUD can prevent complications. Patients suffering from AUD can further decompensate due to the effects of AUD on multiple co-morbidities.

Understanding the effect of AUD on each specific organ system can help diagnose the etiology of the deterioration to allow for optimal treatment and intervention. Further research to understand the development of AUD and the direct relationship between psychiatric illness and AUD can assist in the overall prevention of AUD.

References

1. National Institute on Alcohol Abuse and Alcoholism. Understanding alcohol use disorder. 2023. https://www.niaaa.nih.gov/publications/brochures-and-fact-sheets/understanding-alcohol-use-disorder
2. National Institute on Alcohol Abuse and Alcoholism. Alcohol use disorder comparison between DSM. 2023. https://www.niaaa.nih.gov/publications/brochures-and-fact-sheets/alcohol-use-disorder-comparison-between-dsm
3. Substance Abuse and Mental Health Services Administration. Treatment episode data set. 2020. https://www.samhsa.gov/data/quick-statistics-results?qs_type=teds&state=United%20States&year=2020&type=Admissions&view=full
4. World Health Organization. Global status report on alcohol and health 2018. 2018. www.who.int/substance_abuse/publications/global_alcohol_report/en/
5. Carvalho AF, Heilig M, Perez A, Probst C, Rehm J. Alcohol use disorders. Lancet. 2019;394(10200):781–92.
6. Moss M, Burnham EL. Alcohol abuse in the critically ill patient. Lancet. 2006;368(9554):2231–42.
7. Day E, Daly C. Clinical management of the alcohol withdrawal syndrome. Addiction. 2022;117(3):804–14.
8. Schuckit MA. Recognition and management of withdrawal delirium (delirium tremens). N Engl J Med. 2014;371(22):2109–13.
9. Martínez N, Pintado MC. Substance withdrawal in ICU environment. Oncol Crit Care. 2020:1913–33.
10. Tiberio P, Prendergast N, Mcverry BJ, Wilson JE, Jackson JC, Pandharipande P, Ely EW, Girard TD. Associations between alcohol and illicit drug use and sedative exposure during critical illness. In: TP19. TP019 Quality, process, and outcomes in acute and critical care. American Thoracic Society; 2021. p. A1708.
11. Sanvisens A, Zuluaga P, Fuster D, Rivas I, Tor J, Marcos M, Chamorro AJ, Muga R. Long-term mortality of patients with an alcohol-related Wernicke–Korsakoff syndrome. Alcohol Alcohol. 2017;52(4):466–71.
12. Helle AC, Watts AL, Trull TJ, Sher KJ. Alcohol use disorder and antisocial and borderline personality disorders. Alcohol Res: Curr Rev. 2019;40:1.
13. Castillo-Carniglia A, Keyes KM, Hasin DS, Cerdá M. Psychiatric comorbidities in alcohol use disorder. Lancet Psychiatry. 2019;6(12):1068–80.
14. Rehm J. The risks associated with alcohol use and alcoholism. Alcohol Res Health. 2011;34(2):135.
15. Husain K, Ansari RA, Ferder L. Alcohol-induced hypertension: mechanism and prevention. World J Cardiol. 2014;6(5):245.
16. Helali J, Park S, Ziaeian B, Han JK, Lankarani-Fard A. Thiamine and heart failure: challenging cases of modern-day cardiac beriberi. Mayo Clinic Proceedings: Innovations, Quality & Outcomes. 2019;3(2):221–5.
17. Andersson C, Schou M, Gustafsson F, Torp-Pedersen C. Alcohol intake in patients with cardiomyopathy and heart failure: consensus and controversy. Circulation. Heart Failure. 2022;15(8):e009459.

18. Voskoboinik A, Prabhu S, Ling LH, Kalman JM, Kistler PM. Alcohol and atrial fibrillation: a sobering review. J Am Coll Cardiol. 2016;68(23):2567–76.
19. Voskoboinik A, Kalman JM, De Silva A, Nicholls T, Costello B, Nanayakkara S, Prabhu S, Stub D, Azzopardi S, Vizi D, Wong G. Alcohol abstinence in drinkers with atrial fibrillation. N Engl J Med. 2020;382(1):20–8.
20. De Wit M, Best AM, Gennings C, Burnham EL, Moss M. Alcohol use disorders increase the risk for mechanical ventilation in medical patients. Alcohol Clin Exp Res. 2007;31(7):1224–30.
21. Mehta AJ. Alcoholism and critical illness: a review. World J Care Med. 2016;5(1):27.
22. Scanlan MF, Roebuck T, Little PJ, Naughton MT. Effect of moderate alcohol upon obstructive sleep apnoea. Eur Respir J. 2000;16(5):909–13.
23. Taveira KV, Kuntze MM, Berretta F, de Souza BD, Godolfim LR, Demathe T, De Luca CG, Porporatti AL. Association between obstructive sleep apnea and alcohol, caffeine and tobacco: a meta-analysis. J Oral Rehabil. 2018;45(11):890–902.
24. Burgos-Sanchez C, Jones NN, Avillion M, Gibson SJ, Patel JA, Neighbors J, Zaghi S, Camacho M. Impact of alcohol consumption on snoring and sleep apnea: a systematic review and meta-analysis. Otolaryngology–Head Neck Surg. 2020;163(6):1078–86.
25. Bode C, Bode JC. Alcohol's role in gastrointestinal tract disorders. Alcohol Health Res World. 1997;21(1):76.
26. Clemens DL, Wells MA, Schneider KJ, Singh S. Molecular mechanisms of alcohol associated pancreatitis. World J Gastrointest Pathophysiol. 2014;5(3):147.
27. Yadav D, Papachristou GI, Whitcomb DC. Alcohol-associated pancreatitis. Gastroenterol Clin N Am. 2007;36(2):219–38.
28. Horwich BH, Leven E, Winters AC, Pourmand K. The evolving paradigm of alcohol-associated hepatitis and lreliver transplantation. Clin Liver Dis. 10:2.
29. Gustot T, Jalan R. Acute-on-chronic liver failure in patients with alcohol-related liver disease. J Hepatol. 2019;70(2):319–27.
30. Bernal W, Wendon J. Acute liver failure. N Engl J Med. 2013;369(26):2525–34.
31. Laleman W, Verbeke L, Meersseman P, Wauters J, Van Pelt J, Cassiman D, Wilmer A, Verslype C, Nevens F. Acute-on-chronic liver failure: current concepts on definition, pathogenesis, clinical manifestations and potential therapeutic interventions. Expert Rev Gastroenterol Hepatol. 2011;5(4):523–37.
32. Pitts TO, Van Thiel DH. Disorders of the serum electrolytes, acid-base balance, and renal function in alcoholism. In: Recent developments in alcoholism: combined alcohol and drug abuse typologies of alcoholics the withdrawal syndrome renal and electrolyte consequences; 1986. p. 311–39.
33. Pitts TO, Van Thiel DH. Disorders of divalent ions and vitamin D metabolism in chronic alcoholism. In: Recent developments in alcoholism: combined alcohol and drug abuse typologies of alcoholics the withdrawal syndrome renal and electrolyte consequences; 1986. p. 357–77.
34. Thiele TE, Navarro M, Sparta DR, Fee JR, Knapp DJ, Cubero I. Alcoholism and obesity: overlapping neuropeptide pathways? Neuropeptides. 2003;37(6):321–37.
35. Bahji A, Mazhar MN, Hudson CC, Nadkarni P, MacNeil BA, Hawken E. Prevalence of substance use disorder comorbidity among individuals with eating disorders: a systematic review and meta-analysis. Psychiatry Res. 2019;273:58–66.
36. Baliunas DO, Taylor BJ, Irving H, Roerecke M, Patra J, Mohapatra S, Rehm J. Alcohol as a risk factor for type 2 diabetes: a systematic review and meta-analysis. Diabetes Care. 2009;32(11):2123–32.
37. Rehm J, Anderson P, Kanteres F, Parry CD, Samokhvalov AV, Patra J. Alcohol, social development and infectious disease. Toronto: Centre for Addiction and Mental Health; 2009.
38. Simet SM, Sisson JH. Alcohol's effects on lung health and immunity. Alcohol Res. 2015;37(2):199.
39. Nelson S, Kolls JK. Alcohol, host defence and society. Nat Rev Immunol. 2002;2(3):205–9.
40. Rehm J, Gmel GE Sr, Gmel G, Hasan OS, Imtiaz S, Popova S, Probst C, Roerecke M, Room R, Samokhvalov AV, Shield KD. The relationship between different dimensions of alcohol use and the burden of disease—an update. Addiction. 2017;112(6):968–1001.

41. LoConte NK, Brewster AM, Kaur JS, Merrill JK, Alberg AJ. Alcohol and cancer: a statement of the American Society of Clinical Oncology. J Clin Oncol. 2018;36(1):83–93.
42. American College of Surgeons. National Trauma Data Bank Report 2016. 2016. https://www.facs.org/quality-programs/trauma/quality/national-trauma-data-bank/reports-and-publications/
43. Fabbri A, Marchesini G, Morselli-Labate AM, Rossi F, Cicognani A, Dente M, Iervese T, Ruggeri S, Mengozzi U, Vandelli A. Blood alcohol concentration and management of road trauma patients in the emergency department. J Trauma Acute Care Surg. 2001;50(3):521–8.
44. Chikritzhs T, Livingston M. Alcohol and the risk of injury. Nutrients. 2021;13(8):2777.

Chapter 4
Managing an Opioid-Dependent Patient, Including Acute Opioid Toxicity

Jasper Han and Kunal Karamchandani

Introduction

The rapid rise in opioid abuse and addiction in the United States represents a significant, worsening public health crisis with far-reaching consequences. Opioid-related overdose deaths have surged by 200% since 2000 [1], while hospitals have seen an estimated incidence of 177 out of 100,000 annual emergency department admissions for opioid poisoning [2]. Unsurprisingly, the impact of the opioid epidemic has also extended into the critical care setting, with increases in morbidity and readmission rates [3]. Thus, opioid overuse and abuse, irrespective of etiology, places a significant burden on resources within the healthcare system, particularly on the higher demands within the critical care setting. The common cases of acute overdose toxicity, colloquially referred to as overdose, can be traced to two general sources: prescription opioids and illicit opioid use. Current data from the Centers for Disease Control (CDC) from 1999 to 2017 suggests that deaths from overdose, due to both prescription and illicit opioids, have increased approximately fivefold, with a slightly higher increase seen with illicit opioids [4]. However, there is an intertwined, mutualistic relationship between prescription and heroin overdose deaths; the increase in prescription overdose deaths during a year increased the subsequent year's heroin overdose deaths by a factor of 1.26, whereas, in return, the increase in heroin overdose deaths one year would increase the subsequent year's prescription overdose deaths by a factor of 1.57 [5]. Thus, the prescription of any

J. Han
University of Texas Southwestern Medical School, Dallas, TX, USA

K. Karamchandani (✉)
Department of Anesthesiology and Pain Management, The University of Texas Southwestern Med, Dallas, TX, USA
e-mail: kunal.karamchandani@utsouthwestern.edu

K. Karamchandani, J. E. Grant (eds.), *Substance Use Disorders in Adult Critically Ill Patients*, https://doi.org/10.1007/978-3-031-67069-5_4

opioid requires care and consideration to avoid iatrogenic tolerance, ultimately leading to abuse.

In addition to the life-threatening effects of opioid overdose, opioid tolerance has a wide range of effects specific to the ICU setting. Primarily, pain management in opioid-tolerant patients is difficult, and there is a lack of existing guidelines to direct care in this subset of patients [6]. On the one hand, undertreatment leading to inadequate pain control can result in significant neurologic and psychiatric consequences or withdrawal [7, 8]. At the same time, overtreatment leading to the exacerbation of adverse effects of opioids also carries significant consequences, including gastrointestinal dysfunction complicated by infection, opioid-induced hyperalgesia (OIH), and ultimately opioid toxicity, potentially leading to patient harm [9, 10].

As we discuss below, not only has the opioid epidemic led to an increase in the incidence of ICU admission of opioid dependent patients, but the treatment and management of pain in this vulnerable population is challenging, requiring a fine, balancing act since the consequences of both under- and over-dosing of opioids carry significant implications and long-term results. To explore the impact of opioid usage in critical care, we will discuss two main consequences of opioid dependence in patients presenting to the ICU: acute opioid toxicity and opioid tolerance.

Acute Opioid Toxicity

Acute opioid toxicity is one of the common reasons for an opioid-dependent patient to require ICU-level care. One study looking at ICU admissions from 2009 to 2015 found an average 0.5% increase per month in opioid-related admissions, with a cumulative increase of 34% over 7 years [11]. On the patient side, the monthly mortality rate of those admitted to the ICU with overdose has increased by 0.4%, with a near doubling of ICU deaths related to opioid overdoses from 2009 to 2015 [11]. On the hospital side, there was an adjusted increase of 58% in the average cost per ICU overdose admission during this same time period [11]. These increases suggest that critical care physicians face a mounting challenge in both the incidence and mortality of patients being admitted to the ICU with acute opioid toxicity.

The classic toxidrome, strongly indicative of acute opioid toxicity, consists of miotic pupils, central nervous system (CNS) depression, and a respiratory rate below 12 breaths per minute, with or without evidence of opiate overdose [12]. Other less specific signs include the loss of protective airway reflexes, impaired sensitivity to hypoxemia, and loss of respiratory drive, leading to respiratory arrest and ultimately cardiac arrest [13]. Secondary complications of immobility related to acute opioid toxicity include rhabdomyolysis, myoglobinuric renal failure, and compartment syndrome [13]. In addition to the classic presentation of opioid overdose, certain agents may also have specific side effects, such as methadone, leading to QT prolongation precipitating ventricular tachyarrhythmias [14]. To further confound the clinical picture of opioid toxicity, concurrent intoxication with other non-opioid substances, including antipsychotics, anticonvulsants, ethanol, or other sedative hypnotic agents, may alter the toxidrome, presenting with normal/mydriatic pupils or in the absence of respiratory depression [13]. Earlier findings suggested high (>90%) sensitivity and moderate (>70%) specificity for any one or more of the classic toxidrome, while a recent study in 2016 found lower sensitivity and specificity [15]; this discrepancy may reflect both a varied presentation of different opioid agents or polysubstance use.

While recognition of acute opioid toxicity may be challenging, as mentioned earlier, the management is more straightforward. The mainstay of treatment in a patient suspected of having opioid toxicity is naloxone, a competitive μ opioid-receptor antagonist which reverses the CNS and respiratory effects of opioid intoxication. In acute toxicity, it is administered via the parenteral, intranasal, or pulmonary route for a faster onset of action compared to its negligible bioavailability when administered orally [13]. The dosing of naloxone is empirical since much of the information needed to determine the effective dose is often unknown in an acute setting, including the amount of opioid agent taken, the weight of the patient, and the degree of penetrance into the CNS [16]. The general guideline for empirical naloxone treatment for adults begins with a dose of 0.04 mg, with an increase in dose every 2 minutes to a maximum of 15 mg if there is no response to the treatment, and is titrated to a respiratory rate >12 breaths/minute [13]. If, by 15 mg of naloxone, no response is seen, then other etiologies of respiratory/CNS depression should be considered.

The pharmacokinetics of naloxone are important to consider, as its onset of action is less than 2 minutes when administered intravenously, while its half-life lasts only 20 to 90 minutes [17]. For multiple opioid agents, particularly long-acting opioid agonists used for therapy such as methadone, the agonist effect may persist long after the reversal effects of naloxone subside, causing the patient to relapse into the toxidrome of opioid toxicity. Therefore, vigilance and monitoring are needed even after the administration of a reversal agent, as the offending opioid agent and timeline for recovery are unknown. Naloxone has been traditionally thought to have a highly favorable safety profile and has been advocated to be administered "without compunction." [13] Complications were mainly thought to be those of opioid abstinence, unpleasant but not life threatening [16]. More recently, naloxone has been associated with a dose-dependent, possibly life-threatening, pulmonary edema [18–20]. Additionally, catecholamine release leading to cardiac arrhythmias is a rare but serious adverse effect of naloxone administration. As such, we recommend the above titration of naloxone dosing according to patient response, with vigilant monitoring and supportive care. In addition to naloxone as the mainstay of treatment for acute opioid toxicity, supportive care is needed to maintain ventilation in patients with apnea. In patients with respiratory rates of 12 breaths per minute or less, jaw-thrust and chin-lift maneuvers should be used to increase ventilation and reduce hypercarbia. Positive pressure ventilation via bag-mask devices or mechanical ventilation may be needed for respiratory support in patients with insufficient or ineffective breathing [13, 21]. In the late stages of opioid toxicity, when hemodynamic status is affected, vasopressor or inotrope infusions can be initiated for management [21].

Opioid-Tolerant Patients

Per the Food and Drug Administration (FDA), opioid tolerance is defined as follows: patients receiving, for one week or longer, at least 60 mg oral morphine/day, 25 mcg transdermal fentanyl/hour, 30 mg oral oxycodone/day, 8 mg oral hydromorphone/day, 25 mg oral oxymorphone/day, or an equianalgesic dose of another opioid [22]. As mentioned previously, when patients present to the ICU with chronic opioid use, their substance use can be classified according to the source of the drug as either illicit opioid or long-term prescription opioid usage. The latter include patients taking prescription analgesics for chronic pain as well as patients on medications for OUD (MOUD) for prevention of relapse of OUD. The amount of prescription analgesics sold in 2015 tripled compared to 1999, whereas the incidence of prescription opioid overdose-related deaths increased fourfold between 1999 and 2013 [23, 24]. Since then, the incidence of overdose due to illicit opioid usage has increased to overtake that of prescription opioids [4, 25].

Thus far, we see that illicit opioids and prescription opioids for chronic pain (such as oxycodone, hydrocodone, and morphine) are agents that lead to opioid tolerance. However, even the consumption of MOUD (mainly methadone and buprenorphine/naloxone) can lead to the development of opioid tolerance.

Methadone, a long-acting full-agonist at the μ-opioid receptor, is primarily used as MOUD but is also an option for second-line therapy for chronic pain unresponsive to other forms of opioid treatment [26]. Aside from the other previously mentioned sideeffects, methadone therapy has also been implicated in alterations to pain tolerance with marked hyperalgesia [27]. The other commonly used agent, buprenorphine/naloxone (known by the brand name Suboxone), combines buprenorphine, a partial μ-, full κ-opioid receptor agonist with high affinity, with naloxone, a broad μ-opioid receptor antagonist. As with methadone, this combination medication is primarily used for MOUD but has shown efficacy in pain management and is now being increasingly prescribed as a second-line treatment for pain [28–30]. Also, similar to methadone, buprenorphine/naloxone has pain-modulating effects, but rather than the hyperalgesic effects seen with methadone, buprenorphine/naloxone has shown anti-hyperalgesic effects, potentially reversing the hyperalgesia seen with chronic opioid use [31]. Additional benefits to buprenorphine/naloxone usage compared to other opioids include its enterohepatic metabolism and GI elimination, making it safe to use in patients with renal impairment, as well as a ceiling effect for respiratory depression, preventing the feared complication of respiratory depression complicated by cardiac arrest [32].

The presentation of opioid dependence and tolerance in the ICU involves difficulty in pain management through central sensitization, tolerance, and OIH. Central sensitization occurs when nociceptive pathways are enhanced due to the amplification of pain signals from the nociceptor terminal to dorsal horn neurons, leading to increased action potential output [33]. This process, in the setting of opioid use, heavily involves the glutamate-activated N-methyl-D-aspartate (NMDA) receptor pathway. The NMDA receptor is also implicated in the development of opioid tolerance and OIH [34]. OIH is another side effect of opioid tolerance that complicates the management of pain. This syndrome occurs when the administration and dose escalation of opioids paradoxically worsen rather than improve pain. The molecular mechanism of OIH is not well understood but is thought to be related to neuroplastic changes to the nervous system leading to sensitization of certain pathways, including the glutaminergic pathway and NMDA receptors (as mentioned) [35]. While it can also be found in opioid-naïve patients, it is far more prevalent in patients who have previously been exposed to and are dependent on opioids, particularly in patients with OUD and those suffering from chronic pain [35].

With these complications of opioid dependence in mind, the treatment of acute or acute-on-chronic pain for opioid-tolerant patients in the ICU setting begins with the recognition and assessment of pain. This task is particularly challenging in the ICU setting, as sedation, mechanical ventilation, and critical care conditions confound the verbal, facial, and physiological indicators that could otherwise be used. In a multicenter study, less than half of the ICU providers used pain scales to assess analgesia; the incidence of patients treated for pain was significantly lower than those assessed for pain, suggesting incongruency between providers' decision-making and evaluation of pain [36]. Common methods of pain scoring include the numerical rating scale (NRS), verbal rating scale (VRS), and visual analog scale (VAS) [37]. As patients in the ICU setting are often sedated or encephalopathic and unable to communicate but have intact motor function, behavioral pain scales such as the Critical Care Pain Observation Tool (CPOT) can be used instead [38]. However, studies on the accuracy of these pain scales are inconclusive, without a clear gold standard for validation of diagnostic performance [39, 40]. After assessing the level of pain, the next step in treatment is estimating the daily baseline usage of opioids prior to the current admission. This is best performed by calculating the 24-h oral morphine-equivalent dose to standardize and compare different opioid regimens administered via different routes (oral, transdermal, intravenous). Following this, an equivalent amount of opioid agent should be administered to address the baseline need and supplemented with short-acting opioids for control of the new acute pain. These patients generally need close monitoring to titrate and possibly escalate both the baseline opioid regimen and the short-acting pain control regimen due to chronic use and tolerance.

For ICU patients with previous opioid dependence on pre-existing MOUD, the therapy should be continued in the acute setting, if feasible [41]. The long-acting nature of these medications used for maintenance makes them inappropriate for the management of acute pain, instead requiring supplementation and titration with short-acting opioid analgesics [41]. Due to the development of tolerance, these patients may have added dose requirements, so care must be taken to avoid opioid overdose while trying to achieve sufficient pain control [42–44]. Hemodynamic and respiratory monitoring is crucial as the dosage of short-acting opioids are increased. Another strategy, "opioid rotation", involves switching from one opioid to another. The proposed mechanism behind the effectiveness of this method involves the different interactions of opioids with different receptors (μ, κ, δ, NMDA), leading to varying mechanisms of nociception. Changing the preferential affinity for one type of receptor over another has shown potential to improve analgesia and reduce opioid side effects in chronic pain and possibly in acute settings as well [42, 45]. Other studies suggest that another mechanism behind the beneficial effects of opioid rotation is that the active metabolites of some opioid medications may reduce the analgesic effects of the original agent, and substitution with another opioid medication that has fewer active metabolites may lead to more effective analgesia [46]. Although helpful guidelines for opioid rotation can direct clinician decision-making, caution must be exercised as the evidence supporting this practice is based largely on observational and uncontrolled studies [45, 47].

Opioid-Sparing Options

In the management of opioid-tolerant patients, it is important to consider multimodal pain medication regimens to reduce the use of opioids. Studies have found multimodal pain regimens to be superior to hypnotic-based sedation in the critical care setting [48]. Not only so, the early introduction of adjuvant analgesic agents (non-opioid analgesics) in postoperative patients reduces opioid requirement and side effects, as well as decreased pain scores soon after surgery [49]. The various non-opioid adjuncts are summarized in Table 4.1.

NMDA Antagonists

Opioids influence NMDA receptors in addition to the μ, κ, and δ opioid receptors. The mechanisms of opioid tolerance and OIH are thought to be related to NMDA receptor hyperactivity [50]. Medications that interact with the NMDA receptors are effective in modulating pain. Ketamine is an antagonist at the NMDA receptor, also with lesser effects at the cholinergic, aminergic, and opioid receptor pathways. For pain management, it is generally used for chronic cancer, neuropathic, or postsurgical pain; however, it has also been shown to be noninferior to opioids for the control of acute pain [51]. Furthermore, as an adjunct, it also has an opioid-sparing effect for postsurgical patients [52]. Other benefits of ketamine includes minimal respiratory depression compared to opioids as well as a modest antidepressant effect [50, 53, 54]. It does, however, have side effects such as nausea, vomiting, hallucinations, increased secretions, and myocardial depression in catecholamine-depleted patients, which underscores its routine use for pain management in the ICU. Similar in mechanism to ketamine is dextromethorphan, also an NMDA receptor antagonist, commonly used as an antitussive. In addition, it has also found use as an analgesic adjuvant for various surgical procedures and may have some opioid-sparing effects [55]. More research is needed to sufficiently confirm findings of benefit and characterize the role of dextromethorphan in the critical care setting.

Table 4.1 Non-opioid adjuncts for pain management in critically ill patients

Drug class	Medication	Mechanism of action	Duration/ magnitude of opioid sparing effect	Special considerations in critically ill patients
NMDA antagonists	Ketamine, dextromethorphan	Decreases nociceptive and inflammatory pain transmission by antagonism of NMDA receptor	Up to 40% opioid-sparing effect with ketamine, up to 24 h with dextromethorphan	Myocardial depression leading to potential cardiovascular collapse in sympathetically depleted patients Delirium, hallucinations, vivid dreams Nausea, vomiting
α-2 agonists	Clonidine, dexmedetomidine	Stimulation of α-2 adrenergic pathways in locus coeruleus along with systemic antihypertensive effects	Up to 24 h, greater effect seen with dexmedetomidine	Bradycardia and hypotension
Gabapentinoids	Gabapentin, pregabalin	Decreased release of excitatory neurotransmitters via interactions with α2δ subunits of voltage-gated calcium channels	Opioid-sparing effect likely overestimated but still has some effect, up to 24 h with pregabalin	Dosage adjustment in renal impairment Drowsiness, dizziness, vision change, and imbalance
NSAIDs	Ketorolac, acetaminophen	Central and/or peripheral inhibition of prostaglandin production via COX-1/2 pathways	Up to 24 h with greater efficacy seen in combination of acetaminophen and other NSAIDs	Dosage according to liver (acetaminophen) or kidney (ketorolac) function Ketorolac: risk of GI bleed and platelet dysfunction Acetaminophen: may hide signs of infection, such as fever
SNRIs	Duloxetine	Modulating effect on descending pain pathways in brain and spinal cord	Up to 48 h	Slow onset of action Possible hypertension and tachycardia

(continued)

Table 4.1 (continued)

Drug class	Medication	Mechanism of action	Duration/ magnitude of opioid sparing effect	Special considerations in critically ill patients
TCAs	Amitriptyline	Inhibition of reuptake of norepinephrine and serotonin (similar to SNRIs) and antagonism of spinal NMDA receptors	No clear benefit of use	Decrease in GI motility Drowsiness, dizziness, somnolence Possible hypotension, bradycardia, arrhythmias

NMDA glutamate-activated N-methyl-D-aspartate, *NSAID* non-steroidal anti-inflammatory drugs, *SNRI* serotonin and norepinephrine reuptake inhibitors, *TCA* tricyclic antidepressant

Alpha Adrenergic Agonists

Other medications, such as clonidine and dexmedetomidine, function as α-2 adrenoreceptor agonists to decrease norepinephrine release and enhance parasympathetic activity. The mechanism of the analgesic effects, with possible opioid-sparing benefit, is thought to be due to activity in the locus coerulus while also retaining systemic antihypertensive effects [56]. Because of the possible reduction in opioid requirements, these agents may be considered for opioid weaning, although more data is needed to conclusively support this usage. Compared to clonidine, dexmedetomidine is more potent and has a shorter half-life, allowing for easier titration according to response [53, 57].

Gabapentinoids

Gabapentinoids are a class of drugs that have been traditionally used as antiepileptics but have been generalized to the treatment of neuropathic and chronic pain. The main pathway of action involves interactions between α2δ subunits of voltage-gated calcium channels. The multiple sites of action in the CNS likely account for the alternative and superior pain relief provided [58]. Some studies have shown opioid-sparing effects and demonstrated that gabapentinoids can be used as an adjunct to opioid analgesics [59, 60]. Side effects such as sedation, dizziness, confusion, and potentiation of respiratory depression when used in conjunction with opioids are less ideal for use in critical care.

NSAIDs and Other Medications

Non-steroidal anti-inflammatory drugs (NSAIDs) and acetaminophen, while considered over-the-counter medications, play a role in the multimodal pain regimen for critical care patients. Acetaminophen blocks the central production of prostaglandins, while NSAIDs act on the COX-1 and COX-2 pathways of prostaglandin production in both central and peripheral tissues [61]. Acetaminophen is generally well tolerated, aside from known liver metabolism, and should be added as an adjunct to opioid medications in the setting of acute pain [62]. Masking of fever is a potential limitation of scheduled dosing of acetaminophen, but whether that impacts clinical outcomes is not well established. Although NSAIDs are not commonly used in the ICU setting due to their anti-platelet and gastric side effects, ketorolac is effective as an opioid-sparing agent and has not been associated with increased postoperative bleeding if used judiciously [63].

Other Medications

Psychiatric medications such as duloxetine and tricyclic antidepressants (TCAs) are routinely used for neuropathic pain, similar to gabapetinoids, and have shown varied efficacy as adjuncts to opioid analgesics. Duloxetine is a serotonin and norepinephrine reuptake inhibitor (SNRI) that provides a modulating effect on descending inhibitory pain pathways in the brain and spinal cord. Although studies suggest that it does not provide additional pain relief, graded on a subjective pain scale and compared to placebo, it may lower opioid requirements [64–66]. TCAs, on the other hand, such as amitriptyline, have unclear evidence and often show no difference compared to placebo when used as an adjunct to pain and no reduction in opioid requirements [67, 68]. As such, the current literature does not support the usage of TCAs for the management of pain in the critical care setting.

Regional Anesthesia

While research on the pharmacological opioid-sparing strategies has been progressing, regional analgesia has shown efficacy as a supplement to pharmacological pain management. Regional analgesia (both peripheral and neuraxial), with or without a concurrent opioid analgesic regimen, decreased overall opioid usage and improved perioperative analgesia [69, 70]. Other critical care metrics that showed benefit with regional analgesia include earlier weaning of mechanical ventilation, an earlier return of bowel function after GI surgery, and a reduction in the overall duration of the ICU stay [71, 72].

With peripheral regional analgesia, there are numerous targeted nerve blocks for different surgical procedures and locations of pain. In the upper extremities, a variety of peripheral nerve blocks, including interscalene, supraclavicular brachial plexus, and axillary nerve blocks, all showed benefits including lower pain, decreased opioid consumption, and a longer time to the first analgesic request [73–76]. In the lower extremities, strong evidence supports the finding that a combination of blocks after total knee arthroplasty decreases opioid consumption [77] and provides opioid-sparing effects up to 48 h following procedure [78, 79]. In the proximal structures of the body, such as the abdominal wall, transverse abdominis plane (TAP) blocks offer decreased opioid usage as well as a delayed time to the first analgesic request [80, 81]. These blocks are particularly useful in patients with abdominal incisional pain, commonly seen in the critical care setting following trauma or other surgical procedures. Aside from peripheral blocks, central, neuraxial blocks (thoracic and lumbar epidural analgesia) have been shown to reduce opioid exposure and tolerance, as well as pulmonary morbidity, in addition to the benefits mentioned above [71, 72, 82, 83]. Of note, neuraxial anesthesia is relatively contraindicated in patients on long-term anticoagulant therapy due to the risk of causing spinal hematomas leading to spinal cord ischemia; however, for prophylactic anticoagulation, as commonly seen in the ICU, the epidural catheter can be placed before anticoagulation administration and then continued throughout the duration of prophylaxis [84]. While regional analgesia has shown promising results as part of the multimodal pain regimen, some findings suggest a short-term benefit in pain or opioid reduction but no clear protection against persistent opioid use in the long-term [85–87]. There are also certain cases of rebound pain after regional analgesia [51], possibly further increasing the opioid requirement. For the most part, however, regional analgesia has demonstrated efficacy in non-opioid analgesia and should be considered for multimodal pain management in opioid-tolerant patients.

Future Research and Conclusions

As we have identified in this chapter, the treatment of opioid-dependent patients in the ICU depends on the first step of evaluating pain and opioid requirements, followed by the incorporation of opioid-sparing strategies. Here, we highlight current research potentially leading to future changes in management. As mentioned previously, the methods for assessing pain are largely subjective, with no clear way of standardization, and may not be congruent with one another or with the actual treatment of pain. Additionally, patients in the ICU are often sedated or altogether unresponsive, rendering any scale requiring patient response unusable. Because of this, a standardized, validated scale is needed to direct pain management. In recent years, with the advent of artificial intelligence and machine learning tools, several studies have developed predictive models of future pain in patients with chronic pain [88]. A recent review found that artificial intelligence-based interventions have a positive effect on pain recognition, prediction, and management in chronic pain [89]. As these results have only been proven for chronic pain, there is a need to extrapolate and validate the findings for acute pain, particularly in the ICU setting.

After pain recognition, treatment with opioid-sparing therapies is important to reduce the opioid burden. Many new drugs that are being studied involve specificity toward one or several targets, for example, monoclonal antibodies. Cannabinoids are a class of drug that is commonly used recreationally and less commonly for medicinal purposes. Their role in anxiety, stress, and chronic pain is known to ameliorate sensory, emotional, and cognitive aspects of pain via the endocannabinoid system [90]. However, the usefulness of exogenous cannabinoids in stress-induced hyperalgesia and their opioid-sparing effects for patients in the ICU are not well known [90, 91]. Additionally, the inflammasome and toll-like receptor (TLR) activation pathways have been implicated to affect the response to tissue injury and opioids, affecting both the initial response to analgesia as well as tolerance [92, 93]. This is particularly seen in the setting of critical illness, where patients are in a baseline inflammatory state. TLR activity can be regulated in a stereospecific manner by racemic and isomeric naloxone. Naloxone isomers may be useful to differentiate and modulate the opioid effect on analgesia and the activation of TLRs [94]. Furthermore, inflammasome inhibitors are another area of research in the modulation of nociception. These effects may be particularly useful in managing opioid-induced hyperalgesia and opioid tolerance [95].

With many novel drugs in development, these two that we have mentioned represent only a small portion of the research and development efforts to find non-addictive alternatives to opioids. As these investigations progress, promising drug agents and therapies can be identified for further study and implementation in patient management.

In conclusion, the number of opioid-dependent patients presenting to the ICU is only increasing; interventions during the postoperative or ICU stay may have an important effect on the opioid epidemic. In the treatment of patients with opioid dependence, the first step is recognition either acute opioid toxicity or opioid tolerance; the latter can lead to ineffective pain control and hyperalgesia. The treatment for the former, in general, is naloxone and supportive care, whereas the treatment for the latter involves multimodal methods, including timing or medication rotation as well as adjunctive opioid-sparing therapy. The development of validated pain quantification measures should help with the titration of opioid analgesics, whereas non-addictive alternatives should help to improve treatment and long-term opioid dependence.

References

1. Centers for Disease C, Prevention. Vital signs: overdoses of prescription opioid pain relievers – United States, 199–2008. MMWR Morb Mortal Wkly Rep. 2011;60(43)):1487–92.

2. Weiss AJ, Elixhauser A, Barrett ML, Steiner CA, Bailey MK, O'Malley L. Opioid-Related Inpatient Stays and Emergency Department Visits by State, 2009–2014. Healthcare Cost and Utilization Project (HCUP) Statistical Briefs. 2006. (Updated 2017).
3. Waljee JF, Cron DC, Steiger RM, Zhong L, Englesbe MJ, Brummett CM. Effect of preoperative opioid exposure on healthcare utilization and expenditures following elective abdominal surgery. Ann Surg. 2017;265(4):715–21. https://doi.org/10.1097/SLA.0000000000002117.
4. Prevention CfDCa. 2019 annual surveillance report of drug-related risks and outcomes – United States surveillance special report. Centers for Disease Control and Prevention: U.S. Department of Health and Human Services; 2019.
5. Unick GJ, Rosenblum D, Mars S, Ciccarone D. Intertwined epidemics: national demographic trends in hospitalizations for heroin- and opioid-related overdoses, 1993–2009. PLoS One. 2013;8(2):e54496. https://doi.org/10.1371/journal.pone.0054496.
6. Reichheld AM, Hills-Evans K, Sheehan JK, et al. A national survey of approaches to manage the ICU patient with opioid use disorder. J Crit Care. 2019;54:42–7. https://doi.org/10.1016/j.jcrc.2019.06.032.
7. Jenkins DH. Substance abuse and withdrawal in the intensive care unit. Contemporary issues. Surg Clin North Am. 2000;80(3):1033–53. https://doi.org/10.1016/s0039-6109(05)70112-2.
8. Lewis KS, Whipple JK, Michael KA, Quebbeman EJ. Effect of analgesic treatment on the physiological consequences of acute pain. Am J Hosp Pharm. 1994;51(12):1539–54.
9. Yan Y, Chen Y, Zhang X. The effect of opioids on gastrointestinal function in the ICU. Crit Care. 2021;25(1):370. https://doi.org/10.1186/s13054-021-03793-1.
10. Wang F, Meng J, Zhang L, Roy S. Opioid use potentiates the virulence of hospital-acquired infection, increases systemic bacterial dissemination and exacerbates gut dysbiosis in a murine model of Citrobacter rodentium infection. Gut Microbes. 2020;11(2):172–90. https://doi.org/10.1080/19490976.2019.1629237.
11. Stevens JP, Wall MJ, Novack L, Marshall J, Hsu DJ, Howell MD. The Critical Care Crisis of Opioid Overdoses in the United States. Ann Am Thorac Soc. 2017;14(12):1803–9. https://doi.org/10.1513/AnnalsATS.201701-022OC.
12. Hoffman JR, Schriger DL, Luo JS. The empiric use of naloxone in patients with altered mental status: a reappraisal. Ann Emerg Med. 1991;20(3):246–52. https://doi.org/10.1016/s0196-0644(05)80933-3.
13. Boyer EW. Management of opioid analgesic overdose. N Engl J Med. 2012;367(2):146–55. https://doi.org/10.1056/NEJMra1202561.
14. Butler B, Rubin G, Lawrance A, Batey R, Bell J. Estimating the risk of fatal arrhythmia in patients in methadone maintenance treatment for heroin addiction. Drug Alcohol Rev. 2011;30(2):173–80. https://doi.org/10.1111/j.1465-3362.2010.00213.x.
15. Friedman MS, Manini AF. Validation of Criteria to Guide Prehospital Naloxone Administration for Drug-Related Altered Mental Status. J Med Toxicol. 2016;12(3):270–5. https://doi.org/10.1007/s13181-016-0549-5.
16. Tenenbein M. Continuous naloxone infusion for opiate poisoning in infancy. J Pediatr. 1984;105(4):645–8. https://doi.org/10.1016/s0022-3476(84)80440-0.
17. Berkowitz BA. The relationship of pharmacokinetics to pharmacological activity: morphine, methadone and naloxone. Clin Pharmacokinet. 1976;1(3):219–30. https://doi.org/10.2165/00003088-197601030-00004.
18. Elkattawy S, Alyacoub R, Ejikeme C, Noori MAM, Remolina C. Naloxone induced pulmonary edema. J Community Hosp Intern Med Perspect. 2021;11(1):139–42. https://doi.org/10.1080/20009666.2020.1854417.
19. Al-Azzawi M, Alshami A, Douedi S, Al-Taei M, Alsaoudi G, Costanzo E. Naloxone-induced acute pulmonary edema is dose-dependent: a case series. Am J Case Rep. 2021;22:e929412. https://doi.org/10.12659/AJCR.929412.
20. Schwartz JA, Koenigsberg MD. Naloxone-induced pulmonary edema. Ann Emerg Med. 1987;16(11):1294–6. https://doi.org/10.1016/s0196-0644(87)80244-5.

21. Bowdle TA. Adverse effects of opioid agonists and agonist-antagonists in anaesthesia. Drug Saf. 1998;19(3):173–89. https://doi.org/10.2165/00002018-199819030-00002.
22. Extended-release (ER) and long-acting (LA) opioid analgesics: Risk Evaluation and Mitigation Strategy (REMS). 2012.
23. Reuben DB, Alvanzo AA, Ashikaga T, et al. National Institutes of Health Pathways to Prevention Workshop: the role of opioids in the treatment of chronic pain. Ann Intern Med. 2015;162(4):295–300. https://doi.org/10.7326/M14-2775.
24. Rudd RA, Aleshire N, Zibbell JE, Gladden RM. Increases in Drug and opioid overdose deaths – United States, 2000–2014. MMWR Morb Mortal Wkly Rep. 2016;64(50–51):1378–82. https://doi.org/10.15585/mmwr.mm6450a3.
25. Rudd RA, Seth P, David F, Scholl L. Increases in drug and opioid-involved overdose deaths – United States, 2010–2015. MMWR Morb Mortal Wkly Rep. 2016;65(50–51):1445–52. https://doi.org/10.15585/mmwr.mm655051e1.
26. Davis MP, Walsh D. Methadone for relief of cancer pain: a review of pharmacokinetics, pharmacodynamics, drug interactions and protocols of administration. Support Care Cancer. 2001;9(2):73–83. https://doi.org/10.1007/s005200000180.
27. Doverty M, White JM, Somogyi AA, Bochner F, Ali R, Ling W. Hyperalgesic responses in methadone maintenance patients. Pain. 2001;90(1–2):91–6. https://doi.org/10.1016/s0304-3959(00)00391-2.
28. Rosen K, Gutierrez A, Haller D, Potter JS. Sublingual buprenorphine for chronic pain: a survey of clinician prescribing practices. Clin J Pain. 2014;30(4):295–300. https://doi.org/10.1097/AJP.0b013e318298ddad.
29. Raffa RB, Haidery M, Huang HM, et al. The clinical analgesic efficacy of buprenorphine. J Clin Pharm Ther. 2014;39(6):577–83. https://doi.org/10.1111/jcpt.12196.
30. Pergolizzi J, Boger RH, Budd K, et al. Opioids and the management of chronic severe pain in the elderly: consensus statement of an International Expert Panel with focus on the six clinically most often used World Health Organization Step III opioids (buprenorphine, fentanyl, hydromorphone, methadone, morphine, oxycodone). Pain Pract. 2008;8(4):287–313. https://doi.org/10.1111/j.1533-2500.2008.00204.x.
31. Koppert W, Ihmsen H, Korber N, et al. Different profiles of buprenorphine-induced analgesia and antihyperalgesia in a human pain model. Pain. 2005;118(1–2):15–22. https://doi.org/10.1016/j.pain.2005.06.030.
32. Khanna IK, Pillarisetti S. Buprenorphine – an attractive opioid with underutilized potential in treatment of chronic pain. J Pain Res. 2015;8:859–70. https://doi.org/10.2147/JPR.S85951.
33. Latremoliere A, Woolf CJ. Central sensitization: a generator of pain hypersensitivity by central neural plasticity. J Pain. 2009;10(9):895–926. https://doi.org/10.1016/j.jpain.2009.06.012.
34. Mao J, Sung B, Ji RR, Lim G. Chronic morphine induces downregulation of spinal glutamate transporters: implications in morphine tolerance and abnormal pain sensitivity. J Neurosci. 2002;22(18):8312–23. https://doi.org/10.1523/JNEUROSCI.22-18-08312.2002.
35. Lee M, Silverman SM, Hansen H, Patel VB, Manchikanti L. A comprehensive review of opioid-induced hyperalgesia. Pain Physician. 2011;14(2):145–61.
36. Payen JF, Chanques G, Mantz J, et al. Current practices in sedation and analgesia for mechanically ventilated critically ill patients: a prospective multicenter patient-based study. Anesthesiology. 106(4):687–95; quiz 891–2. https://doi.org/10.1097/01.anes.0000264747.09017.da.
37. Hjermstad MJ, Fayers PM, Haugen DF, et al. Studies comparing Numerical Rating Scales, Verbal Rating Scales, and Visual Analogue Scales for assessment of pain intensity in adults: a systematic literature review. J Pain Symptom Manag. 2011;41(6):1073–93. https://doi.org/10.1016/j.jpainsymman.2010.08.016.
38. Barr J, Fraser GL, Puntillo K, et al. Clinical practice guidelines for the management of pain, agitation, and delirium in adult patients in the Intensive Care Unit: executive summary. Am J Health Syst Pharm. 2013;70(1):53–8. https://doi.org/10.1093/ajhp/70.1.53.

39. Zhai Y, Cai S, Zhang Y. The diagnostic accuracy of critical care pain observation Tool (CPOT) in ICU patients: a systematic review and meta-analysis. J Pain Symptom Manag. 2020;60(4):847–856 e13. https://doi.org/10.1016/j.jpainsymman.2020.06.006.
40. Li MMJ, Ocay DD, Larche CL, et al. Validation of the Critical-Care Pain Observation Tool (CPOT) in pediatric patients undergoing orthopedic surgery. Can J Pain. 2023;7(1):2156332. https://doi.org/10.1080/24740527.2022.2156332.
41. Mehta V, Langford RM. Acute pain management for opioid dependent patients. Anaesthesia. 2006;61(3):269–76. https://doi.org/10.1111/j.1365-2044.2005.04503.x.
42. Mercadante S, Portenoy RK. Opioid poorly-responsive cancer pain. Part 2: basic mechanisms that could shift dose response for analgesia. J Pain Symptom Manag. 2001;21(3):255–64. https://doi.org/10.1016/s0885-3924(00)00236-0.
43. Scimeca MM, Savage SR, Portenoy R, Lowinson J. Treatment of pain in methadone-maintained patients. Mt Sinai J Med. 2000;67(5–6):412–22.
44. Mercadante S, Portenoy RK. Opioid poorly-responsive cancer pain. Part 3. Clinical strategies to improve opioid responsiveness. J Pain Symptom Manag. 2001;21(4):338–54. https://doi.org/10.1016/s0885-3924(01)00250-0.
45. Fine PG, Portenoy RK. Ad Hoc Expert Panel on Evidence R, Guidelines for Opioid R. Establishing "best practices" for opioid rotation: conclusions of an expert panel. J Pain Symptom Manag. 2009;38(3):418–25. https://doi.org/10.1016/j.jpainsymman.2009.06.002.
46. Smith MT. Neuroexcitatory effects of morphine and hydromorphone: evidence implicating the 3-glucuronide metabolites. Clin Exp Pharmacol Physiol. 2000;27(7):524–8. https://doi.org/10.1046/j.1440-1681.2000.03290.x.
47. Quigley C. Opioid switching to improve pain relief and drug tolerability. Cochrane Database Syst Rev. 2004;(3):CD004847. https://doi.org/10.1002/14651858.CD004847.
48. Ehieli E, Yalamuri S, Brudney CS, Pyati S. Analgesia in the surgical intensive care unit. Postgrad Med J. 2017;93(1095):38–45. https://doi.org/10.1136/postgradmedj-2016-134047.
49. Zhao H, Yang S, Wang H, Zhang H, An Y. Non-opioid analgesics as adjuvants to opioid for pain management in adult patients in the ICU: a systematic review and meta-analysis. J Crit Care. 2019;54:136–44. https://doi.org/10.1016/j.jcrc.2019.08.022.
50. Mion G, Villevieille T. Ketamine pharmacology: an update (pharmacodynamics and molecular aspects, recent findings). CNS Neurosci Ther. 2013;19(6):370–80. https://doi.org/10.1111/cns.12099.
51. Lavand'homme P. Rebound pain after regional anesthesia in the ambulatory patient. Curr Opin Anaesthesiol. 2018;31(6):679–84. https://doi.org/10.1097/ACO.0000000000000651.
52. Jouguelet-Lacoste J, La Colla L, Schilling D, Chelly JE. The use of intravenous infusion or single dose of low-dose ketamine for postoperative analgesia: a review of the current literature. Pain Med. 2015;16(2):383–403. https://doi.org/10.1111/pme.12619.
53. Kumar K, Kirksey MA, Duong S, Wu CL. A review of opioid-sparing modalities in perioperative pain management: methods to decrease opioid use postoperatively. Anesth Analg. 2017;125(5):1749–60. https://doi.org/10.1213/ANE.0000000000002497.
54. Costi S, Van Dam NT, Murrough JW. Current status of Ketamine and related therapies for mood and anxiety disorders. Curr Behav Neurosci Rep. 2015;2(4):216–25. https://doi.org/10.1007/s40473-015-0052-3.
55. King MR, Ladha KS, Gelineau AM, Anderson TA. Perioperative dextromethorphan as an adjunct for postoperative pain: a meta-analysis of randomized controlled trials. Anesthesiology. 2016;124(3):696–705. https://doi.org/10.1097/ALN.0000000000000950.
56. Jamadarkhana S, Gopal S. Clonidine in adults as a sedative agent in the intensive care unit. J Anaesthesiol Clin Pharmacol. 2010;26(4):439–45.
57. Wang JG, Belley-Cote E, Burry L, et al. Clonidine for sedation in the critically ill: a systematic review and meta-analysis. Crit Care. 2017;21(1):75. https://doi.org/10.1186/s13054-017-1610-8.

58. Bannister K, Qu C, Navratilova E, et al. Multiple sites and actions of gabapentin-induced relief of ongoing experimental neuropathic pain. Pain. 2017;158(12):2386–95. https://doi.org/10.1097/j.pain.0000000000001040.
59. Mishriky BM, Waldron NH, Habib AS. Impact of pregabalin on acute and persistent postoperative pain: a systematic review and meta-analysis. Br J Anaesth. 2015;114(1):10–31. https://doi.org/10.1093/bja/aeu293.
60. Lam DMH, Choi SW, Wong SSC, Irwin MG, Cheung CW. Efficacy of pregabalin in acute postoperative pain under different surgical categories: a meta-analysis. Medicine (Baltimore). 2015;94(46):e1944. https://doi.org/10.1097/MD.0000000000001944.
61. Vanegas H, Vazquez E, Tortorici V. NSAIDs, opioids, cannabinoids and the control of pain by the central nervous system. Pharmaceuticals (Basel). 2010;3(5):1335–47. https://doi.org/10.3390/ph3051335.
62. Mariano ER, Dickerson DM, Szokol JW, et al. A multisociety organizational consensus process to define guiding principles for acute perioperative pain management. Reg Anesth Pain Med. 2022;47(2):118–27. https://doi.org/10.1136/rapm-2021-103083.
63. Firriolo JM, Nuzzi LC, Schmidtberg LC, Labow BI. Perioperative ketorolac use and postoperative hematoma formation in reduction mammaplasty: a single-surgeon experience of 500 consecutive cases. Plast Reconstr Surg. 2018;142(5):632e–8e. https://doi.org/10.1097/PRS.0000000000004828.
64. Bedin A, Caldart Bedin RA, Vieira JE, Ashmawi HA. Duloxetine as an analgesic reduces opioid consumption after spine surgery. Clin J Pain. 2017;33(10):865–9.
65. YaDeau JT, Brummett CM, Mayman DJ, et al. Duloxetine and subacute pain after knee arthroplasty when added to a multimodal analgesic regimen: a randomized, placebo-controlled, triple-blinded trial. Anesthesiology. 2016;125(3):561–72. https://doi.org/10.1097/ALN.0000000000001228.
66. Castro-Alves LJ, Oliveira de Medeiros AC, Neves SP, et al. Perioperative duloxetine to improve postoperative recovery after abdominal hysterectomy: a prospective, randomized, double-blinded, placebo-controlled study. Anesth Analg. 2016;122(1):98–104. https://doi.org/10.1213/ANE.0000000000000971.
67. Vahedi P, Salehpour F, Aghamohammadi D, et al. Single dose preemptive amitriptyline reduces postoperative neuropathic pain after lumbar laminectomy and discectomy: a randomized placebo-controlled clinical trial. Neurosurg Q. 2010;20(3):151–8. https://doi.org/10.1097/WNQ.0b013e3181ebce15.
68. Kerrick JM, Fine PG, Lipman AG, Love G. Low-dose amitriptyline as an adjunct to opioids for postoperative orthopedic pain: a placebo-controlled trial. Pain. 1993;52(3):325–30. https://doi.org/10.1016/0304-3959(93)90166-M.
69. Richman JM, Liu SS, Courpas G, et al. Does continuous peripheral nerve block provide superior pain control to opioids? A meta-analysis. Anesth Analg. 2006;102(1):248–57. https://doi.org/10.1213/01.ANE.0000181289.09675.7D.
70. Liu SS, Strodtbeck WM, Richman JM, Wu CL. A comparison of regional versus general anesthesia for ambulatory anesthesia: a meta-analysis of randomized controlled trials. Anesth Analg. 2005;101(6):1634–42. https://doi.org/10.1213/01.ANE.0000180829.70036.4F.
71. Guay J, Nishimori M, Kopp SL. Epidural local anesthetics versus opioid-based analgesic regimens for postoperative gastrointestinal paralysis, vomiting, and pain after abdominal surgery: a Cochrane review. Anesth Analg. 2016;123(6):1591–602. https://doi.org/10.1213/ANE.0000000000001628.
72. Popping DM, Elia N, Van Aken HK, et al. Impact of epidural analgesia on mortality and morbidity after surgery: systematic review and meta-analysis of randomized controlled trials. Ann Surg. 2014;259(6):1056–67. https://doi.org/10.1097/SLA.0000000000000237.
73. Ryu T, Kil BT, Kim JH. Comparison between ultrasound-guided supraclavicular and interscalene brachial plexus blocks in patients undergoing arthroscopic shoulder surgery: a prospective, randomized, parallel study. Medicine (Baltimore). 2015;94(40):e1726. https://doi.org/10.1097/MD.0000000000001726.

74. McCartney CJ, Brull R, Chan VW, et al. Early but no long-term benefit of regional compared with general anesthesia for ambulatory hand surgery. Anesthesiology. 2004;101(2):461–7. https://doi.org/10.1097/00000542-200408000-00028.
75. Ilfeld BM, Morey TE, Wright TW, Chidgey LK, Enneking FK. Continuous interscalene brachial plexus block for postoperative pain control at home: a randomized, double-blinded, placebo-controlled study. Anesth Analg. 2003;96(4):1089–95. https://doi.org/10.1213/01.ANE.0000049824.51036.EF.
76. Chan VW, Peng PW, Kaszas Z, et al. A comparative study of general anesthesia, intravenous regional anesthesia, and axillary block for outpatient hand surgery: clinical outcome and cost analysis. Anesth Analg. 2001;93(5):1181–4. https://doi.org/10.1097/00000539-200111000-00025.
77. Terkawi AS, Mavridis D, Sessler DI, et al. Pain management modalities after total knee arthroplasty: a network meta-analysis of 170 randomized controlled trials. Anesthesiology. 2017;126(5):923–37. https://doi.org/10.1097/ALN.0000000000001607.
78. Karlsen AP, Wetterslev M, Hansen SE, Hansen MS, Mathiesen O, Dahl JB. Postoperative pain treatment after total knee arthroplasty: a systematic review. PLoS One. 2017;12(3):e0173107. https://doi.org/10.1371/journal.pone.0173107.
79. Paul JE, Arya A, Hurlburt L, et al. Femoral nerve block improves analgesia outcomes after total knee arthroplasty: a meta-analysis of randomized controlled trials. Anesthesiology. 2010;113(5):1144–62. https://doi.org/10.1097/ALN.0b013e3181f4b18.
80. Ma N, Duncan JK, Scarfe AJ, Schuhmann S, Cameron AL. Clinical safety and effectiveness of transversus abdominis plane (TAP) block in post-operative analgesia: a systematic review and meta-analysis. J Anesth. 2017;31(3):432–52. https://doi.org/10.1007/s00540-017-2323-5.
81. Ilfeld BM, Morey TE, Wang RD, Enneking FK. Continuous popliteal sciatic nerve block for postoperative pain control at home: a randomized, double-blinded, placebo-controlled study. Anesthesiology. 2002;97(4):959–65. https://doi.org/10.1097/00000542-200210000-00031.
82. Capdevila M, Ramin S, Capdevila X. Regional anesthesia and analgesia after surgery in ICU. Curr Opin Crit Care. 2017;23(5):430–9. https://doi.org/10.1097/MCC.0000000000000440.
83. De Pinto M, Dagal A, O'Donnell B, Stogicza A, Chiu S, Edwards WT. Regional anesthesia for management of acute pain in the intensive care unit. Int J Crit Illn Inj Sci. 2015;5(3):138–43. https://doi.org/10.4103/2229-5151.164917.
84. Rowlingson JC, Hanson PB. Neuraxial anesthesia and low-molecular-weight heparin prophylaxis in major orthopedic surgery in the wake of the latest American Society of Regional Anesthesia guidelines. Anesth Analg. 2005;100(5):1482–8. https://doi.org/10.1213/01.ANE.0000148683.54686.0F.
85. Sun EC, Bateman BT, Memtsoudis SG, Neuman MD, Mariano ER, Baker LC. Lack of association between the use of nerve blockade and the risk of postoperative chronic opioid use among patients undergoing total knee arthroplasty: evidence from the Marketscan database. Anesth Analg. 2017;125(3):999–1007. https://doi.org/10.1213/ANE.0000000000001943.
86. Mueller KG, Memtsoudis SG, Mariano ER, Baker LC, Mackey S, Sun EC. Lack of association between the use of nerve blockade and the risk of persistent opioid use among patients undergoing shoulder arthroplasty: evidence from the Marketscan database. Anesth Analg. 2017;125(3):1014–20. https://doi.org/10.1213/ANE.0000000000002031.
87. Ladha KS, Patorno E, Liu J, Bateman BT. Impact of perioperative epidural placement on postdischarge opioid use in patients undergoing abdominal surgery. Anesthesiology. 2016;124(2):396–403. https://doi.org/10.1097/ALN.0000000000000952.
88. Goldstein P, Ashar Y, Tesarz J, Kazgan M, Cetin B, Wager TD. Emerging clinical technology: application of machine learning to chronic pain assessments based on emotional body maps. Neurotherapeutics. 2020;17(3):774–83. https://doi.org/10.1007/s13311-020-00886-7.

89. Zhang M, Zhu L, Lin SY, et al. Using artificial intelligence to improve pain assessment and pain management: a scoping review. J Am Med Inform Assoc. 2023;30(3):570–87. https://doi.org/10.1093/jamia/ocac231.
90. Woodhams SG, Chapman V, Finn DP, Hohmann AG, Neugebauer V. The cannabinoid system and pain. Neuropharmacology. Sep 15 2017;124:105–20. https://doi.org/10.1016/j.neuropharm.2017.06.015.
91. Ueda M, Iwasaki H, Wang S, et al. Cannabinoid receptor type 1 antagonist, AM251, attenuates mechanical allodynia and thermal hyperalgesia after burn injury. Anesthesiology. 2014;121(6):1311–9. https://doi.org/10.1097/ALN.0000000000000422.
92. Ciotu CI, Fischer MJM. Novel analgesics with peripheral targets. Neurotherapeutics. 2020;17(3):784–825. https://doi.org/10.1007/s13311-020-00937-z.
93. Martyn JAJ, Mao J, Bittner EA. Opioid tolerance in critical illness. N Engl J Med. 2019;380(4):365–78. https://doi.org/10.1056/NEJMra1800222.
94. Hutchinson MR, Shavit Y, Grace PM, Rice KC, Maier SF, Watkins LR. Exploring the neuroimmunopharmacology of opioids: an integrative review of mechanisms of central immune signaling and their implications for opioid analgesia. Pharmacol Rev. 2011;63(3):772–810. https://doi.org/10.1124/pr.110.004135.
95. Boriushkin E, Wang JJ, Li J, Bhatta M, Zhang SX. p58(IPK) suppresses NLRP3 inflammasome activation and IL-1beta production via inhibition of PKR in macrophages. Sci Rep. 2016;6:25013. https://doi.org/10.1038/srep25013.

Chapter 5
The Critical Conundrum: Balancing Pain and Opioid Use in Critical Illness

Mary L. Jarzebowski and Morgan Laney

Abbreviations

CIRCI	Critical illness-related corticosteroid insufficiency
GI	Gastrointestinal
HPA	Hypothalamic pituitary axis
ICU	Intensive care unit
ICUAW	ICU acquired weakness
IOWS	Iatrogenic opioid withdrawal syndrome
NPOU	New persistent opioid use
NRS	Numerical rating scale
OIH	Opioid-induced hyperalgesia
OIRD	Opioid-induced respiratory depression
OMME	Oral morphine milligram equivalents
OWS	Opioid withdrawal syndrome
PICS	Post-intensive care syndrome
PTSD	Post-traumatic stress disorder

M. L. Jarzebowski (✉)
Department of Anesthesiology, Pain, and Perioperative Medicine, Henry Ford Health, Detroit, MI, USA
e-mail: mjarzeb1@hfhs.org

M. Laney
Department of Anesthesiology, Corewell Health William Beaumont University Hospital, Royal Oak, MI, USA

K. Karamchandani, J. E. Grant (eds.), *Substance Use Disorders in Adult Critically Ill Patients*, https://doi.org/10.1007/978-3-031-67069-5_5

Introduction

Critical illness is a broad term that encompasses myriad underlying diagnoses, each of which has the potential to cause pain and discomfort to the patient. Surgery and invasive procedures are common in the ICU and further increase the acute pain experienced by critically ill patients. Patients with chronic pain will also need intensive care, with acute conditions potentially worsening an existing pain diagnosis. Despite its many etiologies and morphology, pain is extremely common in the ICU, and undertreating such acute pain is a known source of post-traumatic stress disorder (PTSD) in ICU survivors [1]. Although advances in multimodal analgesia continue, opioids remain the primary treatment modality, with up to 95% of ICU patients receiving opioids during admission [2]. International consensus guidelines recommend frequent evaluation of pain in critical illness [3]. However, such evaluation may be limited by compromised mental status and /or sedation associated with invasive mechanical ventilation. Data suggests that only 42% of mechanically ventilated patients received any pain assessment on day 2 of mechanical ventilation, despite 90% of patients receiving opioids on the same day [4]. Overuse of opioids during critical illness carries its own significant risks to patients. The intensivist prescribing opioids must therefore effectively manage pain, avoiding undertreatment (including iatrogenic withdrawal) while navigating known adverse effects in each patient. This chapter provides a comprehensive review of opioid use in the ICU.

Opioid Withdrawal in the Intensive Care Unit

Opioid withdrawal syndrome (OWS) is a constellation of symptoms that occurs after a decrease in use or complete cessation of opioid medications or after the administration of an opioid antagonist. Symptoms of withdrawal occur within 4 to 48 hours after cessation. Patients may feel irritable and nauseated and experience severe muscle pain, cramping, and diarrhea [5]. Much of the literature on opioid withdrawal in adults uses the definition as stated in the Diagnostic and Statistical Manual, 5th edition. The criteria consider patients to have OWS if they exhibit three or more of the following signs or symptoms within minutes to days after decreasing the dose or stopping use of opioids [6]:

- Agitation or mood dysphoria
- Insomnia
- Muscle pain
- Piloerection
- Yawning
- Rhinorrhea
- Lacrimation
- Mydriasis
- Fever

- Diaphoresis
- Nausea
- Vomiting
- Diarrhea

While OWS is very well studied and understood in the pediatric population, the same does not hold true for adults. There are multiple validated pediatric opioid withdrawal assessment scales and/or tools; however, an adult equivalent remains lacking. Without a standardized assessment tool, diagnosing and studying OWS in adults admitted to the ICU remains challenging [7].

Patients who are admitted to the intensive care unit likely experience OWS in two different scenarios:

1. The patient who uses opioid medications or opioid-containing illicit substances on a chronic basis and does not receive enough opioid medication while admitted to meet their requirements.
2. The opioid-naïve patient who was started on opioids during admission to the hospital (frequently for pain or sedation) and experiences OWS after discontinuation or weaning of those medications. This is known as Iatrogenic Opioid Withdrawal Syndrome (IOWS).

Iatrogenic Opioid Withdrawal Syndrome

A vast majority of ICU patients receive opioid medications during their stay [8, 9]. International consensus guidelines published by the Society of Critical Care Medicine recommend opioid medications, supplemented with opioid-sparing analgesics and non-pharmacologic therapy, as first-line treatment for pain in the ICU [10]. The same guidelines also recommend analgesia-first sedation, defined as the use of opioid pain medication as the initial pharmacologic agent for sedating patients who are receiving mechanical ventilation, with the subsequent addition of traditional sedatives only if needed [8]. The potential benefits of analgesia-first sedation include reduced pain intensity, a shorter duration of mechanical ventilation, and a decreased ICU length of stay [2]. As a result of these guidelines for analgesia and sedation, approximately 85% of critically ill patients will receive opioid medications during their ICU stay, and 15–40% of patients who are maintained on a continuous opioid infusion will develop IOWS during their admission. There are several factors that increase the risk of the development of IOWS [7]:

- Faster rate of infusion weaning
- Patients with a higher body mass index
- Shorter duration of infusion (possibly because a longer duration included the weaning process)
- Concomitant use of a benzodiazepine

Fortunately, opioid withdrawal itself is very rarely a dangerous or life-threatening condition. However, IOWS is unpleasant for the patient, may complicate the treatment plan, and has been shown to increase ICU length of stay [7]. Although there is no duration of opioid exposure that is known to increase the risk for IOWS, providers should consider it in patients who have been taking opioids for >7 days while in the ICU, even if they were not taking them prior to admission. To prevent the development of IOWS, patients should be tapered off opioids when they are no longer needed, rather than stopping abruptly [11]. In general, withdrawal symptoms may begin after 2–3 half-lives of the medication have passed.

If withdrawal symptoms do occur, there are several methods that have been studied to manage IOWS. The first is to restart the opioid medication and slowly taper off over time. The other option is to begin an alpha-2 receptor agonist such as clonidine or dexmedetomidine. While these medications do not target any of the opioid receptors and therefore do not directly decrease withdrawal, they do treat or "mask" the unpleasant symptoms of withdrawal. Finally, there is the option to allow the patients to recover without starting a targeted treatment while solely treating the individual symptoms of withdrawal [5]. This can be achieved with additional medications such as antiemetics, antidiarrheals, and muscle relaxants.

Withdrawal from Chronic Opioid Use While in the ICU

In 2020, the overall national opioid dispensing rate was 43.3 prescriptions per 100 people—the lowest it has been since it peaked at 81.3 prescriptions/100 people in 2012. Over 2 million people in the US suffer from opioid use disorder [12]. The prevalence of opioid use from prescription medication or illicit use means that both dependance and tolerance will be prevalent among patients admitted to the ICU. This presents a challenge to clinicians, making it difficult to adequately treat acute pain experienced in the ICU and placing patients at risk for OWS during admission.

To prevent patients with chronic opioid use from experiencing withdrawal while in the ICU, their daily oral morphine milligram equivalents (OMME) should be calculated correctly and administered using the appropriate route as determined by the treating team (Table 5.1). Additional opioid medication may be supplemented on top of this daily dose as needed for acute pain, procedures, or sedation. Patients taking >30 OMME per day may require up to 4× the dose of opioid medication compared to the opioid-naïve patient for relief from acute pain [13]. Calculating the required dose for patients who use illegal opioid medications is difficult as the dose is commonly unknown and can lead to undertreated pain or OWS.

Table 5.1 Morphine milligram equivalent conversion chart [14]

Types of opioids	MME conversion factors[a]
Common ICU oral opioids	
Hydrocodone	1
Hydromorphone	4
Morphine	1
Opium	1
Oxycodone	1.5
Tramadol	0.1
Common ICU intravenous opioids	
Fentanyl	0.003
Hydromorphone	0.1
Morphine	0.4

[a]When switching routes of administration (PO vs. IV) of opioid medications, tolerance to the drug is the same, and the dose does not need to be altered. When switching between types of opioid medication (e.g., morphine to hydromorphone), the patient may exhibit incomplete opioid receptor cross-tolerance, and medication should be started at 25–50% of the dose while closely monitoring for side effects and increasing as needed for adequate pain control [15]

Considerations in Special Populations

Patients with Intrathecal Pain Pumps

Patients with intrathecal pain pumps should continue intrathecal pain medication if feasible. These infusions are typically high-dose and potent, and patients will often demonstrate high tolerance. This is also important for baclofen-containing solutions. Withdrawal from baclofen can be severe and dangerous [13].

Buprenorphine

If presenting for a planned procedure prior to their admission to the ICU, patients taking buprenorphine may have lowered their buprenorphine dose or stopped the medication altogether, representing concerns that pain may be difficult to treat with a partial μ- agonist present [13]. More contemporary evidence shows that buprenorphine, administered with other full μ-opioid receptor agonists, can produce adequate analgesia for acute pain [16]. Also, buprenorphine itself does have analgesic properties that may be sufficient for perioperative analgesia. For these reasons, new society guidelines recommend that partial opioid agonist therapy should be continued throughout the perioperative period at the same dose as prescribed [17]. There is some evidence that it may be reasonable to decrease the dose for surgical patients in whom adequate pain control is difficult to achieve [18]. Interruption of buprenorphine therapy may increase rates of overdose, relapse, and death [19]. It remains unclear whether the same approach should be used for critically ill patients taking home buprenorphine.

Methadone

Patients may be taking methadone for treatment of chronic pain or for opioid maintenance therapy in addiction. In general, this medication is continued throughout the peri-operative period, avoiding any missed doses. However, methadone can be problematic in the ICU because of its long half-life, unpredictable dosing effects, medication interactions, and side effects. For example, QT prolongation can be exacerbated by the administration of other QT prolonging medications that are commonly used in critical care. For these reasons, methadone is not commonly utilized for acute pain in critical illness; it may be preferrable to trade for another opioid medication or keep the patient's outpatient methadone dose stable and titrate other medications to control acute or new pain [13]. The literature does not easily support an acceptable conversion of methadone into opioid equivalents, as the conversion factor varies depending on the dose [20].

The Consequence of Undertreating Pain During Critical Illness

Pain is often cited as one of the most prevalent and traumatic experiences during patients' ICU stays. Pain is common among ICU patients regardless of the etiology of acute illness or postoperative status, with 51% of all ICU patients reporting rest pain during their ICU admission [21]. Pain during critical illness is also notable for its high severity, as 50% of patients rate ICU pain as moderate to severe at rest and during procedures [21–24]. The location of rest pain seems to be incisional for surgical patients but located in the back and limbs for medical ICU patients [21]. Pain associated with common ICU procedures is also prevalent and reported, especially for chest tube removal, wound drain removal, arterial line insertion, endotracheal suctioning, and even turning in bed [2, 25]. As evidence continues to grow better defining the impact of ICU experiences on patients' recovery from critical illness, the assessment and effective treatment of pain continues to be emphasized to prevent and mitigate significant neurologic and psychiatric sequelae (including post-traumatic stress disorder) associated with ICU survivorship [1].

Although neurologic and psychiatric conditions associated with post-intensive care syndrome (PICS) are common and will be discussed below, other physiologic consequences of undertreated pain may affect all major organ systems (Fig. 5.1) through activation of the sympathetic nervous system, stimulating an acute inflammatory response that may impact the trajectory of illness in myriad ways. It is therefore not surprising that inadequate analgesia is associated with increased hospital morbidity and length of stay, as well as increased cost of hospital stay [26, 27].

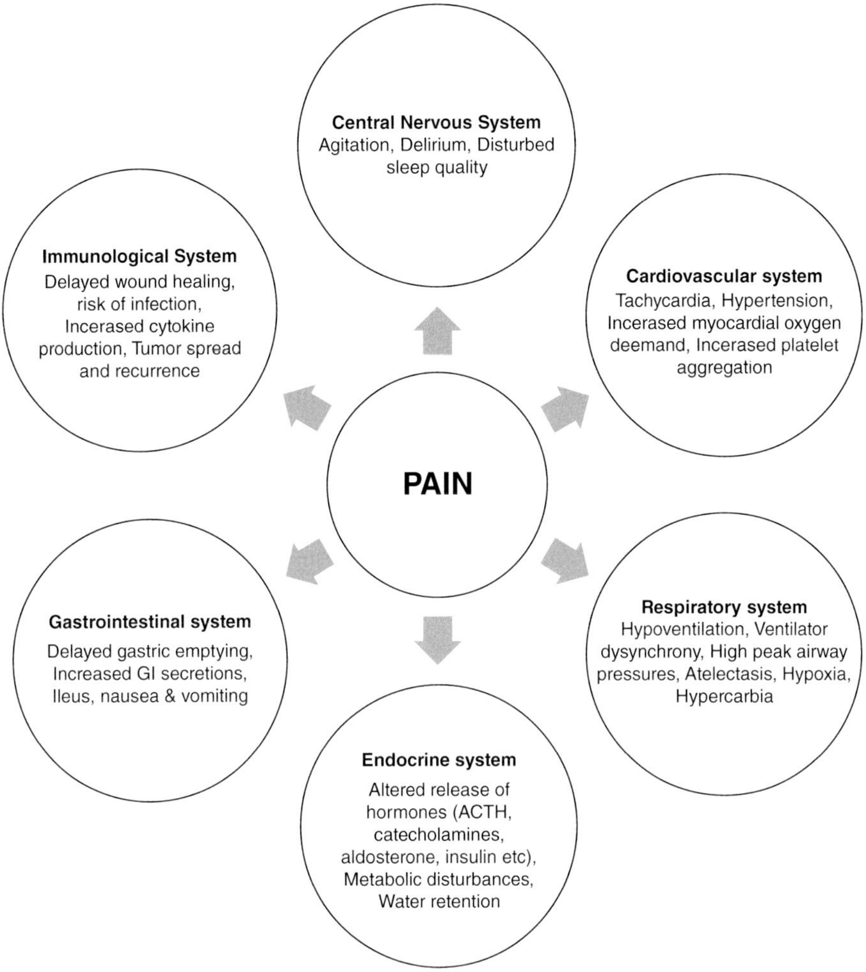

ACTH, adrenocorticotropic hormone; GI, gastrointestinal

Fig. 5.1 Consequence of inadequate pain control. (Reproduced with permission from Karamchandani et al., 2019 [28])

The Scope of Opioid Use in Critically Ill Patients

Given the high incidence of pain associated with acute illness and surgery, as well as the sedative effects desired to facilitate mechanical ventilation, opioid prescribing is almost ubiquitous in critically ill patients [8, 9]. Although granular prescribing practices of opioids in the ICU setting are not well defined, some patterns are noted. In particular, >90% of patients receive opioids during their ICU stay [2, 8, 9]. The average daily opioid consumption (in oral morphine equivalents) for patients receiving mechanical ventilation is 63 mg, which increases to 106 mg daily if mechanical ventilation exceeds seven days in duration [8]. The relative rates of opioid boluses, infusions, and enteral opioids remain unknown. Despite the frequent use of opioids during mechanical ventilation, data suggests that only 20% of patients receiving opioid infusions are assessed with an objective pain scale [9]. It is possible, therefore, that we are overtreating pain during mechanical ventilation and exposing patients to unnecessary harm associated with opioid infusions.

As previously referenced, consensus guideline recommendations from the Society of Critical Care Medicine recommended analgesia-first sedation using an opioid for patients receiving mechanical ventilation prior to initiating a sedative drug [3]. These recommendations reflect the importance of assessing and treating pain to help prevent traumatic experiences during critical illness and minimize delirium. However, the data supporting this practice remains conflicting. Trials that supported the recommendation for opioid-based sedation compared a short-acting opioid (commonly remifentanil) to a benzodiazepine [1, 29, 30]. Given our contemporary knowledge of the poor profile of benzodiazepines in critically ill patients [31–33], it seems logical that such trials demonstrated a shorter duration of mechanical ventilation, less delirium, and a shorter ICU length of stay [29, 34, 35]. However, the superiority of opioid-based sedation over non-benzodiazepine hypnotics (especially propofol and dexmedetomidine) has yet to be demonstrated. Perhaps as a reflection of these guidelines, daily cumulative doses of opioids have been increasing in critically ill patients since 2011 [36].

Adverse Effects of Opioids in ICU Patients

When used in the setting of mechanical ventilation, it is common to administer opioids in the form of an intravenous infusion, which delivers continuous intravenous opioids to the patient. Continuous opioid infusions, although presumed to provide steady pain relief, have been shown in postoperative patients not to significantly improve pain scores over bolused opioid analgesia, despite significantly increasing the total opioid dose administered [37, 38]. Administering opioids as intravenous infusions also alters the drug's pharmacokinetics, leading to potential accumulation of the drug and metabolites, which may increase the likelihood of adverse effects [39]. This is best described using the concept of context-sensitive half-time, which describes the amount of time needed for a drug's serum level to be halved and is dependent on the duration of the infusion [39]. Opioids, such as fentanyl, have particularly long context-sensitive half-times due to their high lipophilicity, and this means the opioid and/or its metabolites may have a clinical effect for many hours after the infusion is stopped. For example, morphine is metabolized to morphine-3-glucuronide, which undergoes renal excretion and may accumulate in patients with renal dysfunction (a common condition in the ICU). Fentanyl undergoes hepatic metabolism, and continuous infusion is known to result in the accumulation and prolongation of its effects [40]. The unique pharmacokinetics of each opioid when delivered as an infusion to a critically ill patient whose drug metabolism is altered by the very nature of their acute illness are unpredictable and the implications of this exposure are unknown.

Also, it is important to note that the primary effect of opioids is analgesia; sedation provided from an opioid is the result of its side effect profile. If an opioid infusion is used as the sole sedative agent, high doses may be needed to achieve a sedation level that is acceptable and comfortable for the patient. This represents a significant opioid exposure, which may increase the likelihood of adverse effects.

Specific Adverse Effects of Opioids

Neurologic

The adverse effects of opioids are well-characterized, impact numerous organ systems (listed in Table 5.2), and have the potential to significantly impact outcomes during critical illness. Opioid administration is now recognized as an independent risk factor for the development of ICU delirium [36], defined as a disturbance of consciousness and cognition that develops over a short period of time and fluctuates over time [41]. The presence of delirium in an ICU patient is associated with a threefold increased risk for 6-month mortality, even after adjusting for confounders [42]. The longer-term impacts of opioids during critical illness on neurologic recovery remain unclear and warrant further investigation, especially when alternative sedating medications exist and are readily available.

Morphine and hydromorphone have been implicated in more specific neurotoxicity due to the accumulation of their active metabolites, morphine-3-glucuronide and hydromorphone-3-glucuronide, respectively [43, 44]. These compounds exert neuroexcitatory effects, which manifest as myoclonus and seizures in their most

Table 5.2 Specific adverse effects of opioids

Domain	Adverse effects
Neurologic	Central nervous system depression Delirium Seizures
Immune	Immunosuppression Nosocomial infection Sepsis
Endocrine	Critical illness-related corticosteroid insufficiency
Respiratory	Opioid-induced respiratory depression
Gastrointestinal	Delayed gastric emptying Nausea and vomiting Constipation Ileus
Pain	New persistent opioid use Hyperalgesia

extreme form [43, 44]. The incidence of neurotoxicity among patients receiving morphine and hydromorphone infusions is unknown.

Respiratory

Opioid-induced respiratory depression (OIRD) is a well-established adverse effect of opioid use, leading to a decreased respiratory drive, hypoxemia, and, if untreated, death. Respiratory depression is common among hospitalized patients, especially among postoperative patients [45], and has been found to significantly increase hospital length of stay [46] and admission costs [47]. More data is needed to evaluate the effects of opioid infusions during mechanical ventilation on the respiratory function of patients following extubation, as residual respiratory depression may present a significant risk to the patient.

Gastrointestinal (GI)

Opioid receptors are present throughout the gastrointestinal tract. Activation of these receptors delays gastric emptying and slows transit through the GI tract in a dose-dependent manner [48, 49], which can manifest as nausea and vomiting, or intolerance to enteral tube feeding in intubated and sedated patients. Data suggests that ICU patients given non-opioid sedation (propofol) have significantly faster gastric emptying times than those given morphine for sedation [50]. Opioids also inhibit the physiologic secretion of electrolytes and water into the intestine, leading to constipation [51]. Constipation is a major issue in critically ill patients, occurring in up to 83% of patients and it is associated with bacterial translocation and prolonged mechanical ventilation [51, 52].

Immune

Opioid-induced immunosuppression has been previously studied in vitro [53, 54], in animal models [55–64], and in human studies [65–68]; however, it was never been studied in critically ill patients, despite having potentially significant effects on the trajectory of a patient's acute illness. The mechanism of this immunosuppression occurs through several potential effects, including inhibition of macrophages and natural killer cells [53, 55–58, 65], disruption of cytokine production [53, 58, 59], impaired migration of macrophages and neutrophils [54, 59, 60], and lymphocyte depletion [64]. These effects on the immune system have translated to clinical significance in several population-based studies of infection risk in patients prescribed chronic opioids, including an increased risk of bacterial pneumonia [69, 70] and an increased risk of serious infection in patients with rheumatoid arthritis [71, 72]. Studies on hospitalized patients, although few, have found an association with higher infection rates when higher-dose intravenous opioids were used in postoperative surgical patients [68] and in burn patients [67]. Impairing immune system competence during critical illness has the potential to significantly impact patient outcomes.

Endocrine

Critically ill patients rely on the endogenous production of cortisol to help respond to their acute illness. Critical illness-related corticosteroid insufficiency (CIRCI) results from dysfunction of the hypothalamic-pituitary-adrenal (HPA) axis during the acute illness, resulting in electrolyte abnormalities, mental status changes, low blood pressure, and possibly worsening shock [73]. Medications have been implicated in this endocrinopathy, most notably etomidate, which was used as a sedative infusion in critically ill patients many decades ago. There is evidence that opioids cause adrenal insufficiency in an outpatient and inpatient setting [74, 75], with impaired cortisol levels seen after even single doses of parenteral opioids [75]. It follows that high-dose opioid infusions may therefore impair the HPA axis during critical illness, although data is lacking on the contribution of opioids to HPA dysfunction in critically ill patients.

New Persistent Opioid Use Following ICU Admission

The ongoing epidemic of opioid use has directed much attention toward identifying opioid exposures that may precipitate an individual's risk for new persistent opioid use (NPOU). Opioid prescription during hospital admission and following surgery have been identified as significantly increasing an individual's risk for NPOU [76, 77]. However, the impact of opioids used during critical illness, and in particular the role of analgesia-first sedation during mechanical ventilation, on the subsequent development of NPOU remains less clear. Also, it is important to question whether new persistent opioid use following critical illness represents a new ongoing pain diagnosis, or perhaps failure to wean opioids aggressively for fear of iatrogenic opioid withdrawal syndrome.

Data suggests that 20%–40% of ICU patients fill an opioid prescription in the week following hospital discharge [78, 79]. Predictors of receiving an opioid prescription at discharge following ICU stay include receipt of mechanical ventilation, surgery, opioids received as an infusion for >4 hours, and sepsis diagnosis [78, 79]. Patients who were discharged with a new opioid prescription following an ICU admission were also found to have had a longer hospital stay following discharge from the ICU, and a higher 30-day mortality than patients who did not receive a new opioid prescription at discharge [79]. Conversely, patients who received a propofol or benzodiazepine infusion during their ICU stay were less likely to be prescribed new opioids at hospital discharge [79]. Further defining potentially modifiable risk factors associated with new opioid prescription at discharge may better inform future research into reducing such prescriptions.

It is important to note that receipt of an opioid prescription at discharge does not necessarily imply consumption of opioids, nor does it imply NPOU. However, longer-term pharmacy records on opioid use after critical illness indicate that 2–10% of patients are still filling opioid prescriptions 6 months after hospital discharge from both medical and surgical intensive care units [78, 80]. Importantly, this data represents only patients who were opioid naïve on hospital admission, therefore identifying those who developed true NPOU. Mean opioid use for these patients remains increased following ICU discharge for at least 24 months, which is the limit of current evidence on the subject [81]. Predictors of continued opioid use 24 months after discharge include older age, lower education level, female sex, prior mental illness diagnosis, prior substance abuse diagnosis, longer ICU length of stay, and receipt of a surgical procedure during ICU admission [78, 81].

Although studies into outpatient opioid prescribing following ICU admission provide important information, the reasons behind ongoing opioid prescribing remain less clear. Some patients will develop new chronic pain following a critical illness [82], but a subset of patients receiving opioids at discharge may represent a failure to actively wean opioids during hospital admission. Indeed, weaning strategies for inpatients who have been receiving high-dose opioids (especially following opioid infusions during mechanical ventilation) have not been well studied. Data suggests that de-escalation to enteral opioids leads to more opioid prescriptions at hospital discharge [83]. However, too abrupt of cessation risks iatrogenic opioid withdrawal. Guidelines for inpatient opioid weaning exist for pediatric patients and recommend reducing the total opioid dose by 10% daily to prevent iatrogenic withdrawal syndrome [84], but data supporting this strategy is lacking, especially in the adult population. More research is needed to further define factors associated with NPOU following critical illness as well as effective opioid weaning strategies for critically ill patients.

Post-ICU Syndrome (PICS)

More than 5 million patients are admitted to US intensive care units annually, spending around 25 million days in the ICU each year as of 2010 [85]. Over the last few decades, ICU survival has increased. Despite the increase in age and comorbidities of patients admitted to the ICU, relative mortality decreased by 35% from 1988 to 2012. As more patients are admitted to and survive their ICU stay, issues unique to ICU survivorship will become increasingly relevant and costly. One such condition is PICS [86]. PICS is a complex disease occurring in ICU survivors which includes impairment in three main components: cognition, mental health, and physical health. These impairments can include a variety of complications, including but not limited to PTSD, cognitive defects, weakness, the inability to complete activities of daily living (ADLs), disordered sleep, and pain [87]. This syndrome represents a significant health burden that will likely increase over time as ICU admissions and discharges continue to rise. This chapter will focus primarily on the pain component of PICS.

Chronic Pain in ICU Survivors

Evidence has consistently demonstrated increased and persistent levels of pain in ICU survivors. Depending on the study, between 14% and 77% of ICU survivors have chronic pain after discharge [82]. Across multiple studies and sources, the most common location for chronic post-ICU pain is the shoulder, followed by back and low extremity pain [82]. A widely accepted definition of persistent post-ICU pain is that which lasts longer than 3–6 months, or longer than a normal period of healing. Importantly, the pain no longer serves a protective function. The major risk factors for the development of chronic post-ICU pain are [88]:

- Acute Respiratory Distress Syndrome
- Acute pain that is present on discharge from the ICU
- Thoracic trauma
- History of chronic pain
- Organ failure
- Sepsis
- Longer ICU length of stay
- Longer duration of mechanical ventilation
- Anxiety and depression after discharge from the ICU
- PTSD

Note that the type of admission (surgical vs. medical) is not a risk factor for the development of post-ICU pain. Interestingly, most studies report a similar occurrence of chronic pain between medical and surgical patients. A difference may be seen in levels of acute pain, with more acute pain in post-surgical patients, but this does not appear to translate to the development of post-ICU pain [88]. This is likely because there is a variety of causes and types of pain that contribute to PICS, most of which are experienced by patients in medical and surgical ICUs.

There are significant consequences of both acute and chronic pain. The physiologic consequences of acute pain have been described above, but particular attention should be given to the psychologic burden associated with acute pain, including anxiety, disrupted sleep, agitation, and delirium [10]. Chronic pain has wide-ranging and devastating complications. It decreases quality of life, interferes with patients' daily activities and productivity, contributes to lost wages, can lead to substance abuse, depression and anxiety, and suicidal ideation, and also leads to a significant increase in the utilization of health care resources [86, 89].

Etiology

Although the precise mechanism of post-ICU pain is not well understood, its etiology is likely similar to other types of chronic pain. In the development of chronic pain, the repeat stimulation of nociceptors leads to hypersensitivity modulation [13]. The typical ICU patient will experience frequent noxious stimuli, including indwelling devices, lines, airways, chest tubes, hardware, and repeat procedures such as thoracentesis and bronchoscopy. Furthermore, many ICU patients are unable to engage in behaviors that would typically serve to alleviate or soothe pain, such as simple actions like repositioning themselves in bed, removing noxious stimuli, or rubbing a painful area [90]. Factors such as sedation, immobility, and impaired communication can make this behavior nearly impossible, leading to increased pain experience. There are many factors that contribute to the transition from acute pain to chronic pain. In a state of chronic inflammation, alterations in nerve pathways occur. There is an increase in afferent nerve firing, central sensitization, and possibly the involvement of the immune response. Current work suggests that the development of persistent pain syndromes may be linked to T-cells as well as auto-antibody-mediated cascades [13].

It remains unknown whether the severity of acute pain experienced in the ICU is related to the likelihood of developing chronic pain. Defining this relationship would help guide how much emphasis should be placed on early and aggressive interventions to reduce pain, including opioids, opioid-sparing analgesics, and non-pharmacologic methods.

Prevention of Chronic Pain

Accurate and reliable assessment of pain in the ICU presents an ongoing challenge, as many patients do not have the ability to report pain due to compromised mental status and sedation associated with mechanical ventilation. Although many validated verbal pain scales (such as the numerical rating scale [NRS]) [91] and non-verbal pain tools exist (such as the Critical-Care Pain Observation Tool [CPOT], and the Face, Legs, Activity, Cry, and Consolability [FLACC]) [92, 93], there is debate regarding the utility of mandated pain assessments in the ICU. Although these assessments have not been shown to decrease the development of post-ICU pain, studies show that frequent assessment of pain leads to less sedation and increased targeted pain management, and therefore remains the standard of care in the ICU [85].

Opioid-sparing analgesics have the advantage of being able to decrease pain with lower opioid use in patients in whom they are safe and tolerated. For example, IV acetaminophen has been shown to decrease morphine use in post-operative patients by up to 46% [13]. Aside from avoiding the numerous side effects of opioids, additional benefit is seen due to the avoidance of opioid-induced hyperalgesia [94]. These medications include acetaminophen, non-steroidal anti-inflammatory medications, ketamine, dexmedetomidine, gabapentin, pregabalin, muscle relaxants, antidepressants, and more. In addition, the Society for Critical Care Medicine recommends four non-pharmacologic interventions to reduce pain: massage therapy, cold therapy, music/sound, and relaxation therapy. Opioid medications are still recommended as first-line therapy for pain in ICU patients that is non-neuropathic in nature, for treatment of pain prior to ICU procedures, and for sedation during mechanical ventilation [10].

Opioid-induced hyperalgesia (OIH) is a concept that has been recognized for many decades and describes a decreased pain tolerance in patients who previously received high-dose opioids [94]. Studies of surgical patients have shown that higher doses of intraoperative opioid correlate with higher pain scores and higher opioid dosing postoperatively [95, 96]. While the mechanisms underlying OIH are unclear, it has the potential to affect the recovery of critically ill patients who received high-dose opioids for both pain and/or sedation. Better data is needed to define the relationship between specific opioid medications, the total cumulative dose used a during critical illness, and the subsequent development of chronic pain.

Management of Post-ICU Syndrome

The management of PICS is multifaceted, and research into effective treatments is still needed. Most importantly, attention should be paid to the prevention of PICS. ICU liberation bundles should be utilized, and focus paid to early ventilator weaning and liberation. As discussed earlier, the longer duration of mechanical ventilation is a major risk factor for PICS, and as such, ventilator weaning strategies are an important part of prevention. Early mobilization and physical therapy, especially in mechanically ventilated patients, go along with this as well. ICU-acquired muscle weakness (ICUAW) is known to impair survival, physical function, and reduce the quality of life. For this reason, rehabilitation and early mobilization can and should be utilized to improve outcomes and reduce pain [97, 98]. There are some sources suggesting that very early physical rehab may be one of the most promising ways to prevent PICS and that beginning physical rehab while still in the ICU is both safe and effective in terms of improving mobility, strength, and days alive out of hospital [95]. Although this does improve muscle strength, there are systematic reviews that show no benefit from early mobilization and rehab as it relates to quality of life and mortality [97]. The use of ICU diaries may reduce PTSD in ICU survivors and their supporting family members [87].

The prognosis and outcome of PICS are not yet well known, as this is a developing area of focus within critical care medicine. There are studies examining the trajectory of chronic pain after ICU discharge with widely variable results. The literature indicates that some post-ICU pain will decrease by 7 months, while other studies show increasing pain beyond 1 year following discharge, and still others indicate relatively stable pain scores for the first year [82]. It is likely that pain trajectories vary based on the etiology of post-ICU pain. A better understanding of post-ICU pain phenotypes may be helpful in identifying effective treatment.

The treatment of PICS and its associated pain should involve early identification and multidisciplinary care. A barrier to this approach is the lack of a cohesive, broadly accepted PICS screening tool. The Healthy Aging Brain Care-Monitor Self Report, originally developed by dementia experts, shows promise for this use [99]. For patients determined to be at risk for or showing signs of PICS, appropriate care should include extensive discharge planning, post-ICU clinics, peer support groups, survivorship programs, access to psychologists and therapy, physical and occupational therapy, and patient and family education.

Post-ICU clinics are intended to recognize ICU-related impairments and provide the correct therapeutic support. The advantage to this model of management is that it is specific to ICU survivors and can be run by critical care providers who are familiar with the unique needs of this patient population. Post-ICU clinics are widely accepted in the United Kingdom but are still gaining support in the United States. Vanderbilt University opened an ICU Recovery Center (ICU-RC) in 2012 that was modeled after multidisciplinary cancer survivor clinics with the hope of addressing the ICU survivorship issues they noted in their patients and families; these issues have since collectively become known as PICS [100]. The results of this study performed at the Vanderbilt ICU-RC indicate this is a feasible and effective method to maximize recovery in the post-ICU discharge period.

PICS and its associated pain remain an area with opportunity for significant improvement, with the goal of maximizing recovery after an ICU stay, minimizing the detrimental effects of the ICU, and reducing the burden on the health care system.

Conclusion

Opioids remain the cornerstone of acute pain management during critical illness. The impact of opioids on both the trajectory of critical illness and the development of chronic pain following ICU discharge remains unclear. Overuse of opioids may precipitate acute adverse effects during admission, hyperalgesia, and new persistent opioid use following discharge. Underuse may lead to suboptimal pain control during admission, higher rates of PTSD in ICU survivors, and an increased likelihood of developing new chronic pain. As critical care continues to evolve, emphasis is now placed on recovery after a critical illness. Defining the role of opioids and finding effective alternatives in critical illness should be a priority to maximize each patient's analgesia and recovery.

References

1. Jackson JC, Pandharipande PP, Girard TD, Brummel NE, Thompson JL, Hughes CG, et al. Depression, post-traumatic stress disorder, and functional disability in survivors of critical illness in the BRAIN-ICU study: a longitudinal cohort study. Lancet Respir Med. 2014;2(5):369–79.
2. Payen JF, Chanques G, Mantz J, Hercule C, Auriant I, Leguillou JL, et al. Current practices in sedation and analgesia for mechanically ventilated critically ill patients: a prospective multicenter patient-based study. Anesthesiology. 2007;106(4):687–95; quiz 891–2.
3. Devlin JW, Skrobik Y, Gélinas C, Needham DM, Slooter AJC, Pandharipande PP, et al. Clinical practice guidelines for the prevention and management of pain, agitation/seda-

tion, delirium, immobility, and sleep disruption in adult patients in the ICU. Crit Care Med. 2018;46(9):e825–e73.

4. Payen JF, Bosson JL, Chanques G, Mantz J, Labarere J, Investigators D. Pain assessment is associated with decreased duration of mechanical ventilation in the intensive care unit: a post Hoc analysis of the DOLOREA study. Anesthesiology. 2009;111(6):1308–16.
5. Sevarino K. Opioid withdrawal in adults: clinical manifestations, course, assessment and diagnosis. In: Saxon A, Friedman M, editors. UpToDate: Wolters Kluwer; 2022.
6. American Psychiatric Association. Diagnostic and statistical manual of mental disorders: DSM-5-TR. 5th, text revision ed. Washington, DC: American Psychiatric Association Publishing; 2022. p. lxix, 1050 pages.
7. Lamey PS, Landis DM, Nugent KM. Iatrogenic opioid withdrawal syndromes in adults in intensive care units: a narrative review. J Thorac Dis. 2022;14(6):2297–308.
8. Wunsch H, Kahn JM, Kramer AA, Rubenfeld GD. Use of intravenous infusion sedation among mechanically ventilated patients in the United States. Crit Care Med. 2009;37(12):3031–9.
9. Burry LD, Williamson DR, Perreault MM, Rose L, Cook DJ, Ferguson ND, et al. Analgesic, sedative, antipsychotic, and neuromuscular blocker use in Canadian intensive care units: a prospective, multicentre, observational study. Can J Anaesth. 2014;61(7):619–30.
10. Barr J, Fraser GL, Puntillo K, Ely EW, Gélinas C, Dasta JF, et al. Clinical practice guidelines for the management of pain, agitation, and delirium in adult patients in the intensive care unit. Crit Care Med. 2013;41(1):263–306.
11. Roberts PR, Todd SR. Society of critical care medicine. Comprehensive critical care: adult. 2nd ed. Mount Prospect: Society of Critical Care Medicine; 2017. p. xii, 600 pages.
12. US Opioid Dispensing Rate Maps Center for Disease Control and Prevention2021 [updated November 10, 2021]. Available from: https://www.cdc.gov/drugoverdose/rxrate-maps/index.html
13. Trentman T. Faust's anesthesiology review. 5th ed. St. Louis: Elsevier; 2019, pages cm p.
14. Services CfMaM. Opioid oral Morphine Equivalent (MME) Conversion Factors table for prescription drug coverage. US Department of Health and Human Services; 2020.
15. Dowell D, Haegerich TM, Chou R. CDC guideline for prescribing opioids for chronic pain – United States, 2016. JAMA. 2016;315(15):1624–45.
16. Macintyre PE, Russell RA, Usher KA, Gaughwin M, Huxtable CA. Pain relief and opioid requirements in the first 24 hours after surgery in patients taking buprenorphine and methadone opioid substitution therapy. Anaesth Intensive Care. 2013;41(2):222–30.
17. Kohan L, Potru S, Barreveld AM, Sprintz M, Lane O, Aryal A, et al. Buprenorphine management in the perioperative period: educational review and recommendations from a multisociety expert panel. Reg Anesth Pain Med. 2021;46(10):840–59.
18. Quaye A, Potter K, Roth S, Acampora G, Mao J, Zhang Y. Perioperative continuation of buprenorphine at low-moderate doses was associated with lower postoperative pain scores and decreased outpatient opioid dispensing compared with buprenorphine discontinuation. Pain Med. 2020;21(9):1955–60.
19. Warner NS, Warner MA, Cunningham JL, Gazelka HM, Hooten WM, Kolla BP, et al. A practical approach for the management of the mixed opioid agonist-antagonist buprenorphine during acute pain and surgery. Mayo Clin Proc. 2020;95(6):1253–67.
20. Walker PW, Palla S, Pei BL, Kaur G, Zhang K, Hanohano J, et al. Switching from methadone to a different opioid: what is the equianalgesic dose ratio? J Palliat Med. 2008;11(8):1103–8.
21. Chanques G, Sebbane M, Barbotte E, Viel E, Eledjam JJ, Jaber S. A prospective study of pain at rest: incidence and characteristics of an unrecognized symptom in surgical and trauma versus medical intensive care unit patients. Anesthesiology. 2007;107(5):858–60.
22. Carroll KC, Atkins PJ, Herold GR, Mlcek CA, Shively M, Clopton P, et al. Pain assessment and management in critically ill postoperative and trauma patients: a multisite study. Am J Crit Care. 1999;8(2):105–17.
23. Stanik-Hutt JA, Soeken KL, Belcher AE, Fontaine DK, Gift AG. Pain experiences of traumatically injured patients in a critical care setting. Am J Crit Care. 2001;10(4):252–9.

24. Puntillo KA, Wild LR, Morris AB, Stanik-Hutt J, Thompson CL, White C. Practices and predictors of analgesic interventions for adults undergoing painful procedures. Am J Crit Care. 2002;11(5):415–29; quiz 30–1.
25. Puntillo KA, Max A, Timsit JF, Vignoud L, Chanques G, Robleda G, et al. Determinants of procedural pain intensity in the intensive care unit. The Europain® study. Am J Respir Crit Care Med. 2014;189(1):39–47.
26. Whipple JK, Lewis KS, Quebbeman EJ, Wolff M, Gottlieb MS, Medicus-Bringa M, et al. Analysis of pain management in critically ill patients. Pharmacotherapy. 1995;15(5):592–9.
27. Crippen DW. The role of sedation in the ICU patient with pain and agitation. Crit Care Clin. 1990;6(2):369–92.
28. Karamchandani K, Klick JC, Linskey Dougherty M, Bonavia A, Allen SR, Carr ZJ. Pain management in trauma patients affected by the opioid epidemic: a narrative review. J Trauma Acute Care Surg. 2019;87(2):430–9.
29. Park G, Lane M, Rogers S, Bassett P. A comparison of hypnotic and analgesic based sedation in a general intensive care unit. Br J Anaesth. 2007;98(1):76–82.
30. Agarwal V, O'Neill PJ, Cotton BA, Pun BT, Haney S, Thompson J, et al. Prevalence and risk factors for development of delirium in burn intensive care unit patients. J Burn Care Res. 2010;31(5):706–15.
31. Pandharipande P, Shintani A, Peterson J, Pun BT, Wilkinson GR, Dittus RS, et al. Lorazepam is an independent risk factor for transitioning to delirium in intensive care unit patients. Anesthesiology. 2006;104(1):21–6.
32. Pandharipande PP, Pun BT, Herr DL, Maze M, Girard TD, Miller RR, et al. Effect of sedation with dexmedetomidine vs lorazepam on acute brain dysfunction in mechanically ventilated patients: the MENDS randomized controlled trial. JAMA. 2007;298(22):2644–53.
33. Pandharipande P, Cotton BA, Shintani A, Thompson J, Pun BT, Morris JA, et al. Prevalence and risk factors for development of delirium in surgical and trauma intensive care unit patients. J Trauma. 2008;65(1):34–41.
34. Breen D, Karabinis A, Malbrain M, Morais R, Albrecht S, Jarnvig IL, et al. Decreased duration of mechanical ventilation when comparing analgesia-based sedation using remifentanil with standard hypnotic-based sedation for up to 10 days in intensive care unit patients: a randomised trial [ISRCTN47583497]. Crit Care. 2005;9(3):R200–10.
35. Karabinis A, Mandragos K, Stergiopoulos S, Komnos A, Soukup J, Speelberg B, et al. Safety and efficacy of analgesia-based sedation with remifentanil versus standard hypnotic-based regimens in intensive care unit patients with brain injuries: a randomised, controlled trial [ISRCTN50308308]. Crit Care. 2004;8(4):R268–80.
36. Duprey MS, Dijkstra-Kersten SMA, Zaal IJ, Briesacher BA, Saczynski JS, Griffith JL, et al. Opioid use increases the risk of delirium in critically ill adults independently of pain. Am J Respir Crit Care Med. 2021;
37. Parker RK, Holtmann B, White PF. Patient-controlled analgesia. Does a concurrent opioid infusion improve pain management after surgery? JAMA. 1991;266(14):1947–52.
38. Chen WH, Liu K, Tan PH, Chia YY. Effects of postoperative background PCA morphine infusion on pain management and related side effects in patients undergoing abdominal hysterectomy. J Clin Anesth. 2011;23(2):124–9.
39. Hughes MA, Glass PS, Jacobs JR. Context-sensitive half-time in multicompartment pharmacokinetic models for intravenous anesthetic drugs. Anesthesiology. 1992;76(3):334–41.
40. Breen D, Wilmer A, Bodenham A, Bach V, Bonde J, Kessler P, et al. Offset of pharmacodynamic effects and safety of remifentanil in intensive care unit patients with various degrees of renal impairment. Crit Care. 2004;8(1):R21–30.
41. Association AP. Diagnostic and statistical manual of mental disorders fourth edition, text revision. 2000.
42. Ely EW, Shintani A, Truman B, Speroff T, Gordon SM, Harrell FE, et al. Delirium as a predictor of mortality in mechanically ventilated patients in the intensive care unit. JAMA. 2004;291(14):1753–62.

43. Smith MT. Neuroexcitatory effects of morphine and hydromorphone: evidence implicating the 3-glucuronide metabolites. Clin Exp Pharmacol Physiol. 2000;27(7):524–8.
44. Klimas R, Mikus G. Morphine-6-glucuronide is responsible for the analgesic effect after morphine administration: a quantitative review of morphine, morphine-6-glucuronide, and morphine-3-glucuronide. Br J Anaesth. 2014;113(6):935–44.
45. Khanna AK, Bergese SD, Jungquist CR, Morimatsu H, Uezono S, Lee S, et al. Prediction of opioid-induced respiratory depression on inpatient wards using continuous capnography and oximetry: an international prospective. Observational Trial Anesth Analg. 2020;131(4):1012–24.
46. Urman RD, Seger DL, Fiskio JM, Neville BA, Harry EM, Weiner SG, et al. The burden of opioid-related adverse drug events on hospitalized previously Opioid-free surgical patients. J Patient Saf. 2021;17(2):e76–83.
47. Khanna AK, Saager L, Bergese SD, Jungquist CR, Morimatsu H, Uezono S, et al. Opioid-induced respiratory depression increases hospital costs and length of stay in patients recovering on the general care floor. BMC Anesthesiol. 2021;21(1):88.
48. Heyland DK, Tougas G, King D, Cook DJ. Impaired gastric emptying in mechanically ventilated, critically ill patients. Intensive Care Med. 1996;22(12):1339–44.
49. Yan Y, Chen Y, Zhang X. The effect of opioids on gastrointestinal function in the ICU. Crit Care. 2021;25(1):370.
50. Bosscha K, Nieuwenhuijs VB, Vos A, Samsom M, Roelofs JM, Akkermans LM. Gastrointestinal motility and gastric tube feeding in mechanically ventilated patients. Crit Care Med. 1998;26(9):1510–7.
51. Mostafa SM, Bhandari S, Ritchie G, Gratton N, Wenstone R. Constipation and its implications in the critically ill patient. Br J Anaesth. 2003;91(6):815–9.
52. Banerjee S, Sindberg G, Wang F, Meng J, Sharma U, Zhang L, et al. Opioid-induced gut microbial disruption and bile dysregulation leads to gut barrier compromise and sustained systemic inflammation. Mucosal Immunol. 2016;9(6):1418–28.
53. House RV, Thomas PT, Bhargava HN. In vitro evaluation of fentanyl and meperidine for immunomodulatory activity. Immunol Lett. 1995;46(1-2):117–24.
54. Malik AA, Radhakrishnan N, Reddy K, Smith AD, Singhal PC. Morphine-induced macrophage apoptosis modulates migration of macrophages: use of in vitro model of urinary tract infection. J Endourol. 2002;16(8):605–10.
55. Shavit Y, Ben-Eliyahu S, Zeidel A, Beilin B. Effects of fentanyl on natural killer cell activity and on resistance to tumor metastasis in rats. Dose Timing study Neuroimmunomodul. 2004;11(4):255–60.
56. Beilin B, Martin FC, Shavit Y, Gale RP, Liebeskind JC. Suppression of natural killer cell activity by high-dose narcotic anesthesia in rats. Brain Behav Immun. 1989;3(2):129–37.
57. Shavit Y, Terman GW, Lewis JW, Zane CJ, Gale RP, Liebeskind JC. Effects of footshock stress and morphine on natural killer lymphocytes in rats: studies of tolerance and cross-tolerance. Brain Res. 1986;372(2):382–5.
58. Sacerdote P, Manfredi B, Mantegazza P, Panerai AE. Antinociceptive and immunosuppressive effects of opiate drugs: a structure-related activity study. Br J Pharmacol. 1997;121(4):834–40.
59. Wang J, Barke RA, Charboneau R, Roy S. Morphine impairs host innate immune response and increases susceptibility to Streptococcus pneumoniae lung infection. J Immunol. 2005;174(1):426–34.
60. Wang J, Barke RA, Charboneau R, Schwendener R, Roy S. Morphine induces defects in early response of alveolar macrophages to Streptococcus pneumoniae by modulating TLR9-NF-kappa B signaling. J Immunol. 2008;180(5):3594–600.
61. Roy S, Cain KJ, Charboneau RG, Barke RA. Morphine accelerates the progression of sepsis in an experimental sepsis model. Adv Exp Med Biol. 1998;437:21–31.
62. Hilburger ME, Adler MW, Truant AL, Meissler JJ, Satishchandran V, Rogers TJ, et al. Morphine induces sepsis in mice. J Infect Dis. 1997;176(1):183–8.

63. Breslow JM, Monroy MA, Daly JM, Meissler JJ, Gaughan J, Adler MW, et al. Morphine, but not trauma, sensitizes to systemic Acinetobacter baumannii infection. J Neuroimmune Pharmacol. 2011;6(4):551–65.
64. Zhang EY, Xiong J, Parker BL, Chen AY, Fields PE, Ma X, et al. Depletion and recovery of lymphoid subsets following morphine administration. Br J Pharmacol. 2011;164(7):1829–44.
65. Beilin B, Shavit Y, Hart J, Mordashov B, Cohn S, Notti I, et al. Effects of anesthesia based on large versus small doses of fentanyl on natural killer cell cytotoxicity in the perioperative period. Anesth Analg. 1996;82(3):492–7.
66. Sacerdote P, Bianchi M, Gaspani L, Manfredi B, Maucione A, Terno G, et al. The effects of tramadol and morphine on immune responses and pain after surgery in cancer patients. Anesth Analg. 2000;90(6):1411–4.
67. Schwacha MG, McGwin G, Hutchinson CB, Cross JM, Maclennan PA, Rue LW. The contribution of opiate analgesics to the development of infectious complications in burn patients. Am J Surg. 2006;192(1):82–6.
68. Horn SD, Wright HL, Couperus JJ, Rhodes RS, Smout RJ, Roberts KA, et al. Association between patient-controlled analgesia pump use and postoperative surgical site infection in intestinal surgery patients. Surg Infect. 2002;3(2):109–18.
69. Dublin S, Walker RL, Jackson ML, Nelson JC, Weiss NS, Von Korff M, et al. Use of opioids or benzodiazepines and risk of pneumonia in older adults: a population-based case-control study. J Am Geriatr Soc. 2011;59(10):1899–907.
70. Wiese AD, Griffin MR, Schaffner W, Stein CM, Greevy RA, Mitchel EF, et al. Opioid analgesic use and risk for invasive pneumococcal diseases: a nested case-control study. Ann Intern Med. 2018;168(6):396–404.
71. Wiese AD, Griffin MR, Stein CM, Mitchel EF, Grijalva CG. Opioid analgesics and the risk of serious infections among patients with rheumatoid arthritis: a self-controlled case series study. Arthritis Rheumatol. 2016;68(2):323–31.
72. Wiese AD, Griffin MR, Schaffner W, Stein CM, Greevy RA, Mitchel EF, et al. Long-acting Opioid use and the risk of serious infections: a retrospective cohort study. Clin Infect Dis. 2019;68(11):1862–9.
73. Marik PE, Pastores SM, Annane D, Meduri GU, Sprung CL, Arlt W, et al. Recommendations for the diagnosis and management of corticosteroid insufficiency in critically ill adult patients: consensus statements from an international task force by the American College of Critical Care Medicine. Crit Care Med. 2008;36(6):1937–49.
74. Daniell HW. Opioid contribution to decreased cortisol levels in critical care patients. Arch Surg. 2008;143(12):1147–8.
75. Donegan D, Bancos I. Opioid-induced adrenal insufficiency. Mayo Clin Proc. 2018;93(7):937–44.
76. Calcaterra SL, Yamashita TE, Min SJ, Keniston A, Frank JW, Binswanger IA. Opioid prescribing at hospital discharge contributes to chronic opioid use. J Gen Intern Med. 2016;31(5):478–85.
77. Brummett CM, Waljee JF, Goesling J, Moser S, Lin P, Englesbe MJ, et al. New persistent opioid use after minor and major surgical procedures in US adults. JAMA Surg. 2017;152(6):e170504.
78. Wunsch H, Hill AD, Fu L, Fowler RA, Wang HT, Gomes T, et al. New Opioid use after invasive mechanical ventilation and hospital discharge. Am J Respir Crit Care Med. 2020;202(4):568–75.
79. Tollinche LE, Seier KP, Yang G, Tan KS, Tayban YD, Pastores SM, et al. Discharge prescribing of enteral opioids in opioid naïve patients following non-surgical intensive care: a retrospective cohort study. J Crit Care. 2022;68:16–21.
80. Karamchandani K, Pyati S, Bryan W, Pepin M, Lehman EB, Krishnamoorthy V, et al. New persistent opioid use after postoperative intensive care in US veterans. JAMA Surg. 2019;154(8):778–80.

81. von Oelreich E, Eriksson M, Sjölund KF, Discacciati A, Larsson E, Oldner A. Opioid use after intensive care: a nationwide cohort study. Crit Care Med. 2021;49(3):462–71.
82. Kemp HI, Laycock H, Costello A, Brett SJ. Chronic pain in critical care survivors: a narrative review. Br J Anaesth. 2019;123(2):e372–e84.
83. Kram B, Weigel KM, Kuhrt M, Gilstrap DL. Discharge prescribing of enteral opioids after initiation as a weaning strategy from continuous opioid infusions in the Intensive Care Unit. J Opioid Manag. 2018;14(1):35–42.
84. Playfor S, Jenkins I, Boyles C, Choonara I, Davies G, Haywood T, et al. Consensus guidelines on sedation and analgesia in critically ill children. Intensive Care Med. 2006;32(8):1125–36.
85. Nordness MF, Hayhurst CJ, Pandharipande P. Current perspectives on the assessment and Management of Pain in the intensive care unit. J Pain Res. 2021;14:1733–44.
86. Brown SM, Bose S, Banner-Goodspeed V, Beesley SJ, Dinglas VD, Hopkins RO, et al. Approaches to addressing post-intensive care syndrome among intensive care unit survivors. A narrative review. Ann Am Thorac Soc. 2019;16(8):947–56.
87. Mikkelsen M, Netzer G, Iwashyna T. In: Finlay G, Manaker S, editors. Post-intensive care syndrome (PICS). UpToDate: Wolters Kluwer; 2022.
88. Mäkinen OJ, Bäcklund ME, Liisanantti J, Peltomaa M, Karlsson S, Kalliomäki ML. Persistent pain in intensive care survivors: a systematic review. Br J Anaesth. 2020;125(2):149–58.
89. Hayhurst CJ, Jackson JC, Archer KR, Thompson JL, Chandrasekhar R, Hughes CG. Pain and its long-term interference of daily life after critical illness. Anesth Analg. 2018;127(3):690–7.
90. Johnson J, Al-Dahir S. Chronic post-ICU pain and post-intensive care syndrome. US Pharmacist. 2016;41(3):11–5.
91. Nugent SM, Lovejoy TI, Shull S, Dobscha SK, Morasco BJ. Associations of pain numeric rating scale scores collected during usual care with research administered Patient reported pain outcomes. Pain Med. 2021;22(10):2235–41.
92. Gélinas C, Fillion L, Puntillo KA, Viens C, Fortier M. Validation of the critical-care pain observation tool in adult patients. Am J Crit Care. 2006;15(4):420–7.
93. Manworren RC, Hynan LS. Clinical validation of FLACC: preverbal patient pain scale. Pediatr Nurs. 2003;29(2):140–6.
94. Hayhurst CJ, Durieux ME. Differential Opioid tolerance and opioid-induced hyperalgesia: a clinical reality. Anesthesiology. 2016;124(2):483–8.
95. Salengros JC, Huybrechts I, Ducart A, Faraoni D, Marsala C, Barvais L, et al. Different anesthetic techniques associated with different incidences of chronic post-thoracotomy pain: low-dose remifentanil plus presurgical epidural analgesia is preferable to high-dose remifentanil with postsurgical epidural analgesia. J Cardiothorac Vasc Anesth. 2010;24(4):608–16.
96. Guignard B, Bossard AE, Coste C, Sessler DI, Lebrault C, Alfonsi P, et al. Acute opioid tolerance: intraoperative remifentanil increases postoperative pain and morphine requirement. Anesthesiology. 2000;93(2):409–17.
97. Tipping CJ, Harrold M, Holland A, Romero L, Nisbet T, Hodgson CL. The effects of active mobilisation and rehabilitation in ICU on mortality and function: a systematic review. Intensive Care Med. 2017;43(2):171–83.
98. Berney S, Haines K, Skinner EH, Denehy L. Safety and feasibility of an exercise prescription approach to rehabilitation across the continuum of care for survivors of critical illness. Phys Ther. 2012;92(12):1524–35.
99. Wang S, Allen D, Perkins A, Monahan P, Khan S, Lasiter S, et al. Validation of a new clinical tool for post-intensive care syndrome. Am J Crit Care. 2019;28(1):10–8.
100. Sevin CM, Bloom SL, Jackson JC, Wang L, Ely EW, Stollings JL. Comprehensive care of ICU survivors: development and implementation of an ICU recovery center. J Crit Care. 2018;46:141–8.

Chapter 6
Nicotine Use Disorders: Impact on Critical Illness and Therapeutic Strategies

Victoria Mroz and Zdravka Zafirova

Abbreviations

ALI	Aacute lung injury
ANS	Autonomic nervous system
ARDS	Acute respiratory distress syndrome
BAL	Bronchoalveolar lavage
BIPAP	Bilevel positive airway pressure
CAP	Community-acquired pneumonia
CBD	Cannabinoid
CKD	Chronic kidney disease
COPD	Chronic obstructive pulmonary disease
COVID-19	Coronavirus disease-19
CPAP	Continuous positive airway pressure
CT	Computer tomography
ENDS	Electronic nicotine delivery system
ESR	Erythrocyte sedimentation rate
ESRD	End-stage renal disease
EVALI	E-cigarette and vaping acute lung injury
GABA	Gamma-aminobutyric acid
GERD	Gastroesophageal reflux disease

V. Mroz
Icahn School of Medicine, New York, NY, USA
e-mail: victoria.mroz@icahn.mssm.edu

Z. Zafirova (✉)
Department of Cardiovascular Surgery, Icahn School of Medicine, Mount Sinai Hospital, New York, NY, USA
e-mail: Zdravka.zafirova@mountsinai.org

K. Karamchandani, J. E. Grant (eds.), *Substance Use Disorders in Adult Critically Ill Patients*, https://doi.org/10.1007/978-3-031-67069-5_6

GI	Gastrointestinal
HAP	Hospital-acquired pneumonia
IBD	Inflammatory bowel disease
ICU	Intensive care unit
LES	Lower esophageal sphincter
NTP	Nicotine and tobacco products
NTUD	Nicotine and tobacco use disorder
nAChRs	Nicotinic cholinergic receptors
HIV	Human immunodeficiency virus
PCR	Polymerase chain reaction
PNS	Parasympathetic nervous system
PUD	Peptic ulcer disease
RCC	Renal cell carcinoma
SARS-CoV-2	Severe acute respiratory syndrome coronavirus 2
SCD	Sudden cardiac death
SNS	Sympathetic nervous system
THC	Tetrahydrocannabinol

Introduction

Nicotine and tobacco use disorders (NTUD) have been recognized worldwide as a major public health concern with wide-ranging consequences for both the individuals and the entire society. Nicotine and tobacco products (NTP) pose numerous health risks and are a major cause of preventable morbidity and mortality due to their biochemical effects and their addictive nature, with the development of dependence, tolerance, and withdrawal symptoms upon cessation. Prevalence studies consistently demonstrate the widespread nature of nicotine use disorders. In the United States, the National Survey on Drug Use and Health reported that in 2021, approximately 54.7 million people (19.5%) aged 12 or older used a tobacco product, and 13.2 million people (4.7%) used an e-cigarette or other vaping device to vape nicotine [1]. The costs of healthcare utilization, productivity loss, premature disability, and death due to nicotine-related diseases impose a substantial economic burden on the individual and the population.

Nicotine use has been established as a significant risk factor for the development and progression of critical cardiovascular disease, pulmonary disease, and certain cancers. The health impact has evolved with the emergence of new nicotine electronic delivery systems (ENDS), such as electric cigarettes and vaping devices, which have been associated with similar cardiovascular effects, as well as critical pulmonary complications such as e-cigarette and vaping acute lung injury (EVALI), highlighting the importance of studying the relationship between nicotine use and emerging pulmonary complications.

Neuropsychiatric Alterations

Nicotine stimulates the nicotinic cholinergic receptors (nAChRs) in the central nervous system (cortex, hippocampus, thalamus), the autonomic nervous system (ANS)—sympathetic (SNS) and parasympathetic nervous system (PNS), autonomic ganglia, the neuromuscular junction, the peripheral sensory nerves, the adrenal medulla, immune cells, and gastrointestinal tract. The resulting release of various neurotransmitters, including dopamine, epinephrine, norepinephrine, acetylcholine, serotonin, vasopressin, gamma-aminobutyric acid (GABA), glutamate, and endorphins, triggers a wide range of responses, such as mood modulation, arousal, cognitive and memory improvement, analgesia, appetite suppression, and immune function alterations. Nicotine also upregulates nAchR expression. The increase in the mesolimbic dopamine signaling by nicotine is at the basis of the motivational and rewarding behavior that develops with nicotine exposure and triggers a repetitive cycle of use and dependence [2–5]. With chronic exposure, adaptation of the neural pathways leads to reduced brain reward function and nicotine withdrawal symptoms with abstinence, including bradycardia and gastrointestinal discomfort (suggestive of ANS disruption), depressed mood, decreased arousal, irritability, sleep disturbances, and cognitive deficits including attention, working memory, and episodic memory impairments [3–5]. Nicotine has a negative impact on sleep, and smokers are more likely to experience sleep apnea, sleep disordered breathing, insomnia, and poor sleep quality [3, 4].

In the critical care setting, nicotine withdrawal has been associated with increased agitation, delirium, self-removal of support devices, prolonged ventilator days and intensive care unit (ICU) length of stay, and morbidity [6, 7]. Smoking has been identified as a risk factor for violence in delirious patients [8]. Screening of patients for tobacco use, timing, and amount may aid in predicting the risk of withdrawal. The Fagerström Test for Nicotine Dependence (FTND) and Nicotine Dependence Syndrome Scale (NDSS) can be used as screening tools; however, they have not been validated in the intensive care setting. These patients may have higher sedation and analgesia needs, and medical regimens may need to be adjusted accordingly. Vigilant monitoring for the development of withdrawal, delirium, and related complications is essential to prevent morbidity and mortality. Nicotine replacement therapy has been used in the ICU. However, it has not been proven to consistently reduce withdrawal events; while some trials have suggested the treatment benefit of delirium in smokers in ICU, others have not supported it, and the quality of the data is suboptimal [9, 10]. Some studies have raised concerns regarding increased vasospasm, cardiovascular events, and mortality, while other trials have not demonstrated a negative mortality impact. Therefore, prophylactic use of NRT in the ICU setting cannot be strongly recommended. Therapeutic use in ICU delirium may be considered in select patients with a clear history of current significant NTP use and in whom other causes of delirium have been addressed. It should be individualized, considering the patient's other, particularly cardiovascular, comorbidities.

Cardiovascular Alterations

The cardiovascular effects of nicotine and other tobacco products are linked to activation of the SNS and release of catecholamines, leading to tachycardia, increased contractility, increased vascular resistance, and blood pressure increases [11]. Endothelia dysfunction, altered platelet aggregation, proinflammatory response, oxidative damage, angiogenesis abnormalities, and dyslipidemia have also been demonstrated in chronic tobacco users [11]. These vasoconstrictive, inflammatory, and metabolic effects can be noted after acute exposure and more prominently after chronic prolonged use, contributing to the development and acceleration of atherosclerosis, hypertension, coronary and peripheral vascular artery disease, myocardial infarction, stroke, and arrhythmia [11]. Similar effects on some cardiovascular parameters have been demonstrated in recent studies with nicotine-containing e-cigarettes [12, 13], albeit not with a consistent degree [14]. A study by Alzahrani et al. found that e-cigarette use was independently associated with a higher likelihood of having a heart attack, even after adjusting for traditional cardiovascular risk factors [15]. E-cigarette use contributes to the increased risk of acute cardiac events and chronic cardiovascular disease [16–18].

Nicotine affects the electrical activity of the heart by influencing ion channels and neurotransmitter release, leading to enhanced sympathetic activity, disruption of the balance between SNS and PNS, and prolonged action potential duration [19]. Carbon monoxide and oxidative stress contribute to the arrhythmogenic effects of tobacco [19]. Smokers often exhibit a higher resting heart rate compared to nonsmokers, and these effects can be observed even after a single cigarette. E-cigarettes in tobacco users prolong the ventricular repolarization [20, 21]. Tobacco and e-cigarette use are associated with an increased risk of supraventricular and ventricular arrhythmia, such as atrial fibrillation and ventricular tachyarrhythmias [19–22]. Furthermore, the risk of sudden cardiac death (SCD) in patients with coronary artery disease is significantly higher with tobacco use [23, 24]. A recent meta-analysis indicated a three-fold increase in SCD among current smokers and a 38% increase in former smokers [25]. The majority of the episodes of SCD were due to ventricular tachyarrhythmias [25]. Clinicians should be cognizant of cardiovascular disease in patients who are active or recent users of tobacco products, including e-cigarettes. In the critical care unit, vigilant monitoring for symptoms and signs of acute coronary syndrome, cerebrovascular events, and heart failure should be applied [26]. Continuous electrocardiography monitoring and analysis of the ventricular repolarization are helpful in identifying patients at risk for critical arrhythmia. The QT interval and the corrected QTc interval for heart rate as indices of ventricular repolarization should be a part of the standard monitoring; the Tp-e interval, the peak of the T wave to the end of the T wave, represents only ventricular repolarization and is demonstrated to be a better predictor of ventricular arrhythmias and SCD and should be evaluated particularly in these high-risk patients [19, 27]. Proactive management of atrial and ventricular arrhythmias aims to reduce the cardiovascular morbidity and mortality [27].

Respiratory System Changes

The use of nicotine and tobacco products in the setting of active smoking and in second-hand and prenatal exposure is associated with various pulmonary pathologies, including reactive airway disease (asthma, bronchitis), bronchiectasis, chronic obstructive pulmonary disease (COPD), respiratory tract infections, tuberculosis, lung cancer, acute respiratory distress syndrome (ARDS), and e-cigarette/vaping-associated lung injury (EVALI) [28]. Furthermore, NTUD significantly increases the mortality risk for COPD, asthma, tuberculosis, and lung cancer [28].

The detrimental effects of NTP on the lung stem from direct insult due to the noxious tobacco particles, exogenous oxidative injury, activation of the inflammatory response and endogenous oxidative damage, and DNA alterations [29]. The pro-inflammatory response, via the recruitment and activation of inflammatory cells into the lung, production and upregulation of inflammatory mediators, cellular adhesion molecules, and extracellular matrix components, results in alveolar and endothelia damage and disruption of the repair mechanisms [30, 31]. The cellular alterations, mucosal injury, impaired mucociliary clearance, alveolar destruction, pulmonary fibrosis, and chronic inflammation lead to increased airway reactivity, susceptibility to infections and allergic reactions, and cancerogenic impact, thus contributing to the development and worsening of lung pathologies and a progressive decline in lung function [32]. The use of e-cigarettes and vaping nicotine delivery systems is similarly associated with disruption of the lung immune response, cellular function, and DNA alterations, thus contributing to pulmonary pathology [18, 33, 34]. Smokers are at significantly higher risk of acute exacerbations of pulmonary illness and infectious predisposition, leading to increased rates of ICU admission, morbidity, and mortality. And therefore, there is a heightened focus for critical care providers [35].

In patients with smoking-associated COPD, the decline in lung function and the disease severity progression increases the likelihood of exacerbations and ICU admissions; severe exacerbations are associated with higher mortality rates [36, 37]. Smokers with COPD and asthma are more susceptible to respiratory morbidity, including infections such as community-acquired (CAP) and hospital-acquired pneumonia (HAP), as compared to never smokers [35, 38]. Furthermore, NTUD in patients with CAP is associated with an increase in ICU admission rates, length of stay, need for mechanical ventilation, and mortality [38, 39]. Lung disease exacerbation should be managed proactively with inhaled and systemic pharmacotherapy, including bronchodilators, anti-inflammatory agents, and respiratory support, as per the current guidelines [40–43]. The pathogen profile in smokers may differ from nonsmokers [38]; therefore, along with empiric antimicrobial therapy, microbiological studies should be done in patients admitted to the ICU, to identify the pathogens and guide targeted therapy. Current and former smokers have higher odds of influenza-associated hospital and ICU admission, and deaths compared to never smokers [44]. These high-risk patients should be identified and should be monitored for the development of severe symptoms and the need for advanced respiratory support.

The impact of NTUD on COVID infections has been a focus of multiple investigations and the results have garnered some controversy [45–47]. The variability of the study methodologies, including differentiation between current and former smokers and the inconsistent accounting for the duration and amount of smoking, present challenges in interpreting the data, some of which indicate worse outcomes in current and former smokers with SARS-CoV-2 infections, while others have failed to demonstrate effect difference. Nonetheless, current, and former tobacco use is linked with an increase in severe outcomes from SARS-CoV-2 infections, including hospital and ICU admissions, intubation, and death. Therefore, clinicians should anticipate the severe presentation of COVID infection in smokers and apply the current treatment recommendations proactively in these patients.

E-Cigarette/Vaping-Associated Lung Injury (EVALI)

Electronic nicotine delivery system (ENDS) use has been associated with pulmonary disease, including asthma, chronic lung disease, pneumothorax, and a spectrum of inflammatory lung pathologies—eosinophilic and hypersensitivity pneumonitis, bronchiolitis, pneumonia, diffuse alveolar hemorrhage and EVALI [18, 48, 49]. Centers for disease control and prevention (CDC) published data in 2020, documenting 2807 hospitalizations for EVALI and 68 deaths [50]. While the age range was 13–85, the median age was 24, and 75% of the patients were younger than 35. In patients presenting with an acute lung injury of unclear etiology, a detailed history of NTUD should be sought. Furthermore, patients using ENDS, who present with respiratory and inflammatory symptoms, should be monitored for the development of EVALI. Various inhaled chemical components and mixtures of the ENDS are implicated in the etiology of EVALI, including nicotine, tetrahydrocannabinol (THC), cannabinoid oils (CBD), vitamin E acetate, propylene glycol, diethylene glycol, and medium-chain triglycerides (MCT) [51–53]. The exact etiology remains to be clarified, as multiple components of ENDS alone or in combination may precipitate lung injury. Furthermore, illicit, unregulated ENDS may contain several toxic agents [51, 54]. The pathology of EVALI can demonstrate nonspecific inflammation, diffuse alveolar damage, acute fibrinous pneumonitis, granulomatous pneumonitis and organizing pneumonia [55]. The bronchoalveolar lavage (BAL) of patients with EVALI demonstrates the presence of inflammatory cells such as neutrophils, lymphocytes, and macrophages, specifically lipid-laden macrophages, which can further be identified with an oil red O stain. The lung biopsies of patients and postmortem examinations of the fatal cases reveal focal inflammation, interstitial and peribronchiolar granulomatous pneumonitis, and organizing fibrinous exudates and pneumonia [56]. The resulting alterations in cell signaling, inflammation, oxidative stress, cytotoxicity, and impaired tissue remodeling lead to a disrupted immune response, impaired mucociliary clearance, alterations in pulmonary function tests, and disruption of alveolar gas exchange, as well as increased propensity for superimposed infection.

The clinical presentation of acute to subacute lung injury (ALI) within days to weeks includes respiratory, constitutional, and gastrointestinal involvement. The respiratory symptoms of cough, dyspnea on exertion and at rest, wheezing, chest pain, hemoptysis, and hypoxia are present in nearly all patients and will require respiratory support with supplemental oxygen and noninvasive and invasive mechanical ventilation. Fever, chills, night sweats, fatigue, weight loss, headache, and myalgia are commonly present, as well as gastrointestinal manifestations of nausea, vomiting, and abdominal pain and may precede the respiratory presentation [18, 49, 51]. A case of cardiac arrest as an EVALI presentation has been reported [57]. On examination, increased work of breathing, tachypnea, wheezing, rhonchi, and crackles can be noted, along with fever, tachycardia, hypoxia and hypertension, and pulmonary function test abnormalities. Blood testing demonstrates hypoxemia with respiratory alkalosis and an inflammatory state with leukocytosis, elevated erythrocyte sedimentation rate (ESR), C-reactive protein, and procalcitonin, while rheumatologic serology is negative, as is the infectious testing, in the absence of secondary infection [18, 49, 55, 58, 59]. Testing for common respiratory bacterial and viral pathogens is important, including respiratory and blood cultures, as well as PCR studies. Further targeted microbiological investigation is based on the patients' health risk and environmental background. BAL can aid in the diagnostic evaluation and can be performed; however, it is not required. A preprocedural assessment should be done to evaluate for contraindications as well as whether the BAL may confer significant clinical risk due to precipitating further respiratory compromise or the inability to tolerate sedation due to cardiovascular or neurologic comorbidities.

The diagnostic imaging of EVALI includes chest radiography and computer tomography (CT) and typically demonstrates bilateral symmetric ground-glass opacities with associated septal thickening, characteristic of organizing pneumonia, with subpleural sparing, or predominantly lower lobe consolidation, as well as diffuse centrilobular nodules; rarely, these may represent pulmonary hemorrhage [60]. Additionally, pleural effusions, pneumothorax, and pneumomediastinum may be present [61–63]. The diagnosis of EVALI is based on several criteria [64].

Confirmation of a case of EVALI requires all the following criteria:

- ENDS use in 90 d before symptom onset
- Presence of pulmonary infiltrate on a plain film chest radiograph or ground-glass opacities on a chest CT
- Absence of pulmonary infection on initial work-up: negative respiratory viral panel, influenza PCR/rapid test, urine antigen for Streptococcus pneumoniae and Legionella, HIV-related opportunistic respiratory infections (if indicated), sputum culture, BAL culture, blood culture
- Absence of alternative plausible diagnoses such as cardiac, autoimmune, rheumatologic, or neoplastic processes

The diagnosis of a probable case of EVALI is based on the following:

- ENDS use in 90 d before symptom onset

- Presence of pulmonary infiltrate on a plain film chest radiograph or ground-glass opacities on a chest CT
- Absence of alternative plausible diagnoses such as cardiac, autoimmune, rheumatologic, or neoplastic processes
- Infection not determined to be the sole cause of the underlying lung injury, if infection has not been ruled out (insufficient testing or results) or is identified via culture or PCR

The management of EVALI includes respiratory support, inflammation control, and treatment of superimposed infection [18, 49, 59, 63, 64]. While ambulatory management, with close regular follow-up within 24–48 h, can be considered for a select few mild cases of otherwise healthy patients with maintained oxygenation, most of these patients require hospitalization and intensive monitoring. Early admission to an ICU unit for signs of deterioration and increased oxygen need is advised. The respiratory support needs range from low-flow supplemental oxygen to higher-flow/pressure noninvasive support with a high-flow nasal canula or *continuous positive airway pressure* (CPAP) or bilevel positive airway pressure (BIPAP), and possible escalation to invasive mechanical ventilation and extracorporeal membrane oxygenation intervention [18, 49]. Empiric antimicrobial therapy should be considered in severe cases and further refined based on the infectious testing. Glucocorticosteroids aid in the control of inflammation and should be considered. Their role in improving outcomes in ARDS in general is still not clearly defined, while benefits in specific inflammatory states such as SARS-CoV-2 ALI are more consistently supported by the scientific data. In EVALI, glucocorticoid benefits are suggested by some investigations and may help in the control of severe injury, as well as recovery, and reduce readmissions [18, 59]. However, robust, well-designed clinical trials are lacking, and their use should proceed with caution, particularly in the setting of a significant infection.

Persistent EVALI has necessitated a lung transplant [65].

Investigations of the long-term outcomes from EVALI indicate that clinical and radiographic recovery may require weeks to months, and readmissions and emergency room visits, particularly in patients with pulmonary comorbidities, should be anticipated and a clinical follow-up process should be devised [66–68]. Development or recurrent EVALI and readmissions with continuous use of ENDS are indicated by the clinical data. Considering the young demographic of the ENDS users and EVALI patients, a comprehensive intervention program to ascertain quitting ENDS and recovery from NTUD is an essential public and individual health measure [64, 66–69].

Impact on Infection and Wound Healing

The disruption in the immune response, blood supply, tissue regeneration, and oxidative stress contribute to impaired wound healing and an increased risk of surgical site infections in smokers compared to prior smokers and never smokers; furthermore, some degree of risk remains in patients who have quit NTP [70, 71].

Furthermore, in NTP users with burns, impaired wound healing, a higher intubation rate, and mortality have been demonstrated [71]. Therefore, a heightened focus on the wound prevention and surgical wound care in NTUD patients is required.

Gastrointestinal Alterations

Gastrointestinal (GI) symptoms are prevalent among individuals with NTUD and can affect various aspects of gastrointestinal function. The effects of NTP on the GI system include a decrease in lower esophageal sphincter pressure (LES), impairment of GI motility, an increase in gastric acid secretion and clearance reduction, a reduction in bicarbonate production, as well as an impairment of mucosal blood flow, an alteration of mucosal cellular proliferation, apoptosis, and cellular renewal, and an alteration of the microbiome [72–75]. These effects lead to mucosal damage and impaired regeneration, impaired mucosal immune response, and increased susceptibility to infections, contributing to the development and progression of GI disorders in smokers. Dyspepsia, peptic ulcer disease (PUD), gastroesophageal reflux disease (GERD), and biliary disease are more prevalent in smokers, as are irritable bowel syndrome (IBS) and inflammatory bowel disease (IBD). The impact on IBD is dichotomic, with a higher prevalence of Crohn's disease and a reduced risk of ulcerative colitis. Smokers have an increased risk of Helicobacter pylori infection [72, 76, 77]. ENDS are similarly associated with GI disorder risk, including IBS and dysmotility.

Furthermore, the carcinogenic impact is evident from a multitude of toxic components in cigarette smoke, including the activation of nAChR, alteration of the immune response, formation of DNA adducts, and stimulation of tumor angiogenesis, thus increasing the risk of GI cancers in NTP users. The airway management of a critically ill patient can be impacted by the aforementioned disorders, and their presence should be anticipated and symptoms actively elicited. Precautions to minimize aspiration risk, proactive management of dysmotility, as well as increased awareness regarding the increased risk of bleeding or ischemia, are integral to the best care practices in the ICU.

Endocrine Disorders

Nicotine's impact on glucose homeostasis and insulin sensitivity can contribute to the development of insulin resistance and type 2 diabetes. Studies have shown that nicotine can impair insulin signaling pathways, increase hepatic glucose production, and induce inflammation, all of which can contribute to the pathogenesis of diabetes [78, 79]. Furthermore, nicotine exposure has been associated with an increased risk of diabetes-related complications, such as cardiovascular disease, microvascular disorders (retinopathy, neuropathy, nephropathy), poor glycemic control, and mortality. In the ICU setting, adherence to stringent glucose control intervention is essential to reduce morbidity and mortality, particularly in patients with NTUD.

Nicotine has been shown to interfere with thyroid and corticosteroid hormone synthesis, metabolism, and binding, potentially leading to alterations in thyroid function [80, 81]. Studies have reported an association between NTP and an increased risk of thyroid disorders, such as hypothyroidism, thyroid nodules, and malignancies. Nicotine's impact on thyroid function may be mediated through its effects on the hypothalamic-pituitary-thyroid axis, as well as its potential to promote oxidative stress and inflammation in the thyroid gland. NTPs have been implicated in the development and progression of adrenal gland disorders, specifically primary and secondary adrenal insufficiencies [82, 83]. Nicotine's vasoconstrictive effects and its potential to suppress the hypothalamic-pituitary-adrenal axis may contribute to adrenal dysfunction. The impact of NTP on the development and control of endocrine disorders necessitates targeted testing, monitoring, and management, particularly in critically ill patients, to avoid significant morbidity and mortality.

Renal Pathophysiology

NTP use has been linked, as an independent factor and in conjunction with other medical conditions, to kidney disorders, including chronic kidney disease (CKD), end-stage renal disease (ESRD), nephrolithiasis, and renal cell carcinoma (RCC) [74, 84–86]. NTPs affect the renal blood flow and glomerular filtration rate, oxidative stress, inflammation, and endothelial dysfunction, inducing and exacerbating renal injury. Studies have demonstrated a higher risk of CKD and accelerated disease progression with smoking, as well as increased mortality in CKD [87]. Some investigations have indicated an association between the duration of NTP exposure and CKD and have suggested that smoking cessation may ameliorate the elevated kidney risk. However, a study of lung transplant recipients has demonstrated an increased incidence of CKD in former smokers compared to never smokers [88].

Nicotine's impact on renal blood flow and the urinary system, along with its potential to modify the composition of urine and promote calcium oxalate crystal deposition, may contribute to the development of kidney stones. Several studies have reported a positive association between smoking and the risk of RCC, even for smaller quantities of smoking; additionally, it has a negative impact on overall and disease-specific mortality, as well as on cancer-specific and progression-free survival [89, 90]. Nicotine and other toxic substances in tobacco smoke can enter the bloodstream and accumulate in the kidneys, potentially leading to DNA damage, cellular mutations, and the development of cancerous cells.

E-cigarette use has emerged as a concerning factor in relation to kidney health. Although research on the direct effects of e-cigarettes on the kidneys is limited, the potential harmful renal effects from constituents in e-cigarette aerosols, including nicotine, flavorings, and additives, as well as byproducts from the heating and aerosolization process, contribute to renal damage. Further studies are needed to elucidate the specific mechanisms and long-term consequences of e-cigarette use on kidney health. Due to multiple factors, critically ill patients have a propensity for developing acute kidney injury and for the progression of CKD. NTUD further exacerbates the renal injury risk, and renal protective strategies to avoid further damage are warranted and should be applied in a manner similar to the management of patients with other kidney risk factors [91].

Critically ill patients, actively using NTPs or past users, are susceptible to neurocognitive, cardiovascular, pulmonary, and endocrine disorders and require heightened monitoring and diagnostic and therapeutic interventions to improve health outcomes and reduce healthcare resource utilization. The use of NRT in hospitalized patients who are active NTP users may help reduce withdrawal symptoms. However, in the ICU setting, the prophylactic use of NRT cannot be recommended based on the existing evidence. Signs and symptoms of nicotine withdrawal should be sought but may be challenging to discern. Therapeutic use of NTP should be applied selectively, considering the benefits and the potential risks.

References

1. https://www.samhsa.gov/data/release/2021-national-survey-drug-use-and-health-nsduh-releases
2. Benowitz NL. Pharmacology of nicotine: addiction, smoking-induced disease, and therapeutics. Annu Rev Pharmacol Toxicol. 2009;49:57–71.
3. Valentine G, Sofuoglu M. Cognitive effects of nicotine: recent progress. Curr Neuropharmacol. 2018;16:403–14.
4. Wills L, Ables JL, Braunscheidel KM, Caligiuri SPB, Elayouby KS, Fillinger C, Ishikawa M, Moen JK, Kenny PJ. Neurobiological mechanisms of nicotine reward and aversion. Pharmacol Rev. 2022;74:271–310.
5. Hajdusianek W, Żórawik A, Waliszewska-Prosół M, Poręba R, Gać P. Tobacco and nervous system development and function-new findings 2015–2020. Brain Sci. 2021;11:797.
6. Lucidarme O, Seguin A, Daubin C, Ramakers M, Terzi N, Beck P, Charbonneau P, du Cheyron D. Nicotine withdrawal and agitation in ventilated critically ill patients. Crit Care. 2010;14:R58.
7. Park H, Kim KW, Yoon IY. Smoking cessation and the risk of hyperactive delirium in hospitalized patients: a retrospective study. Can J Psychiatr. 2016;61:643–51.
8. Tachibana M, Inada T, Ichida M, Ozaki N. Risk factors for inducing violence in patients with delirium. Brain Behav. 2021;11:e2276.
9. Ng KT, Gillies M, Griffith DM. Effect of nicotine replacement therapy on mortality, delirium, and duration of therapy in critically ill smokers: a systematic review and meta-analysis. Anaesth Intensive Care. 2017;45:556–61.
10. Kanova M, Tejkalova K, Neiser J, Kula R. Nicotine replacement therapy in surgical patients. Neuro Endocrinol Lett. 2021;42:305–11.
11. Benowitz NL, Burbank AD. Cardiovascular toxicity of nicotine: implications for electronic cigarette use. Trends Cardiovasc Med. 2016;26:515–23.
12. MacDonald A, Middlekauff HR. Electronic cigarettes and cardiovascular health: what do we know so far? Vasc Health Risk Manag. 2019;15:159–74.

13. Gonzalez JE, Cooke WH. Acute effects of electronic cigarettes on arterial pressure and peripheral sympathetic activity in young nonsmokers. Am J Physiol Heart Circ Physiol. 2021;320:H248–55.
14. Haptonstall KP, Choroomi Y, Moheimani R, Nguyen K, Tran E, Lakhani K, Ruedisueli I, Gornbein J, Middlekauff HR. Differential effects of tobacco cigarettes and electronic cigarettes on endothelial function in healthy young people. Am J Physiol Heart Circ Physiol. 2020;319:H547–56.
15. Alzahrani T, Pena I, Temesgen N, Glantz SA. Association between electronic cigarette use and myocardial infarction. Am J Prev Med. 2018;55:455–61.
16. Skotsimara G, Antonopoulos AS, Oikonomou E, Siasos G, Ioakeimidis N, Tsalamandris S, Charalambous G, Galiatsatos N, Vlachopoulos C, Tousouli D. Cardiovascular effects of electronic cigarettes: a systematic review and meta-analysis. Eur J Prev Cardiol. 2019;26:1219–28.
17. Rahman A, Alqaisi S, Alzakhari R, Saith S. Characterization and summarization of the impact of electronic cigarettes on the cardiovascular system: a systematic review and meta-analysis. Cureus. 2023;15:e39528.
18. Rose JJ, Krishnan-Sarin S, Exil VJ, Hamburg NM, Fetterman JL, Ichinose F, Perez-Pinzon MA, Rezk-Hanna M, Williamson E, American Heart Association Council on Cardiopulmonary, Critical Care, Perioperative and Resuscitation, Council on Epidemiology and Prevention, Council on Cardiovascular Radiology and Intervention, Council on Lifestyle and Cardiometabolic Health, Council on Peripheral Vascular Disease, Stroke Council, Council on Arteriosclerosis, Thrombosis and Vascular Biology. Cardiopulmonary impact of electronic cigarettes and vaping products: a scientific statement from the American Heart Association. Circulation. 2023;148:703–28.
19. D'Alessandro A, Boeckelmann I, Hammwhöner M, Goette A. Nicotine, cigarette smoking and cardiac arrhythmia: an overview. Eur J Prev Cardiol. 2012;19:297–305.
20. Ruedisueli I, Lakhani K, Nguyen R, Gornbein J, Middlekauff HR. Electronic cigarettes prolong ventricular repolarization in people who smoke tobacco cigarettes: implications for harm reduction. Am J Physiol Heart Circ Physiol. 2023;324:H821–32.
21. Ip M, Diamantakos E, Haptonstall K, Choroomi Y, Moheimani RS, Nguyen KH, Tran E, Gornbein J, Middlekauff HR. Tobacco and electronic cigarettes adversely impact ECG indexes of ventricular repolarization: implication for sudden death risk. Am J Physiol Heart Circ Physiol. 2020;318:H1176–84.
22. Carll AP, Arab C, Salatini R, Miles MD, Nystoriak MA, Fulghum KL, Riggs DW, Shirk GA, Theis WS, Talebi N, Bhatnagar A, Conklin DJ. E-cigarettes and their lone constituents induce cardiac arrhythmia and conduction defects in mice. Nat Commun. 2022;13:6088.
23. Goldenberg I, Jonas M, Tenenbaum A, Boyko V, Matetzky S, Shotan A, Bezafibrate Infarction Prevention Study Group, et al. Current smoking, smoking cessation, and the risk of sudden cardiac death in patients with coronary artery disease. Arch Intern Med. 2003;163:2301–5.
24. Goldenberg I, Moss AJ, McNitt S, Zareba W, Daubert JP, Hall WJ, Andrews ML, Multicenter Automatic Defibrillator Implantation Trial-II Investigators. Cigarette smoking and the risk of supraventricular and ventricular tachyarrhythmias in high-risk cardiac patients with implantable cardioverter defibrillators. J Cardiovasc Electrophysiol. 2006;17:931–6.
25. Aune D, Schlesinger S, Norat T, Riboli E. Tobacco smoking and the risk of sudden cardiac death: a systematic review and meta-analysis of prospective studies. Eur J Epidemiol. 2018;33:509–21.
26. Aune D, Schlesinger S, Norat T, Riboli E. Tobacco smoking and the risk of heart failure: a systematic review and meta-analysis of prospective studies. Eur J Prev Cardiol. 2019;26:279–88.
27. Ninni S, Layec J, Brigadeau F, Behal H, Labreuche J, Klein C, Schurtz G, Potelle C, Coisne A, Lemesle G, Lamblin N, Klug D, Lacroix D. Incidence and predictors of mortality after an electrical storm in the ICU. Eur Heart J Acute Cardiovasc Care. 2022;11:431–9.
28. Jayes L, Haslam PL, Gratziou CG, Powell P, Britton J, Vardavas C, Jimenez-Ruiz C, Leonardi-Bee J, Tobacco Control Committee of the European Respiratory Society. SmokeHaz: systematic reviews and meta-analyses of the effects of smoking on respiratory health. Chest. 2016;150:164–79.

29. Strzelak A, Ratajczak A, Adamiec A, Feleszko W. Tobacco smoke induces and alters immune responses in the lung triggering inflammation, allergy, asthma and other lung diseases: a mechanistic review. Int J Environ Res Public Health. 2018;15:1033.
30. Bhalla DK, Hirata F, Rishi AK, Gairola CG. Cigarette smoke, inflammation, and lung injury: a mechanistic perspective. J Toxicol Environ Health B Crit Rev. 2009;12:45–64.
31. Faux SP, Tai T, Thorne D, Xu Y, Breheny D, Gaca M. The role of oxidative stress in the biological responses of lung epithelial cells to cigarette smoke. Biomarkers. 2009;14(Suppl 1):90–6.
32. Münzel T, Hahad O, Kuntic M, Keaney JF, Deanfield JE, Daiber A. Effects of tobacco cigarettes, e-cigarettes, and waterpipe smoking on endothelial function and clinical outcomes. Eur Heart J. 2020;41:4057–70.
33. Novelli CE, Higginbotham EJ, Kapanke KA, Webber-Ritchey KJ, Parker CH, Simonovich SD. A systematic review examining the pulmonary effects of electronic vapor delivery systems. J Clin Anesth. 2022;82:110952.
34. Roberts J, Chow J, Trivedi K. Adult-onset asthma associated with E-cigarette use. Curcus. 2021;13:e19190.
35. Lange P, Colak Y, Ingebrigtsen TS, Vestbo J, Marott JL. Long-term prognosis of asthma, chronic obstructive pulmonary disease, and asthma-chronic obstructive pulmonary disease overlap in the Copenhagen City Heart study: a prospective population-based analysis. Lancet Respir Med. 2016;4:454–62.
36. Jo YS. Long-term outcome of chronic obstructive pulmonary disease: a review. Tuberc Respir Dis (Seoul). 2022;85:289–301.
37. Morjaria JB, Campagna D, Caci G, O'Leary R, Polosa R. Health impact of e-cigarettes and heated tobacco products in chronic obstructive pulmonary disease: current and emerging evidence. Expert Rev Respir Med. 2022;16(11–12):1213–26.
38. Crisafulli E, Cillóniz C, Liapikou A, Ferrari M, Busti F, Girelli D, Torres A. Systemic inflammatory response and outcomes in community-acquired pneumonia patients categorized according to the smoking habit or presence of chronic obstructive pulmonary disease. J Clin Med. 2020;9:2884.
39. Yu Y, Liu W, Jiang HL, Mao B. Pneumonia is associated with increased mortality in hospitalized COPD Patients: a systematic review and meta-analysis. Respiration. 2021;100:64–76.
40. Halpin DMG, Criner GJ, Papi A, Singh D, Anzueto A, Martinez FJ, Agusti AA, Vogelmeier CF. Global initiative for the diagnosis, management, and prevention of chronic obstructive lung disease. The 2020 GOLD science committee report on COVID-19 and chronic obstructive pulmonary disease. Am J Respir Crit Care Med. 2021;203(1):24–36.
41. Holguin F, Cardet JC, Chung KF, Diver S, Ferreira DS, Fitzpatrick A, Gaga M, Kellermeyer L, Khurana S, Knight S, McDonald VM, Morgan RL, Ortega VE, Rigau D, Subbarao P, Tonia T, Adcock IM, Bleecker ER, Brightling C, Boulet LP, Cabana M, Castro M, Chanez P, Custovic A, Djukanovic R, Frey U, Frankemölle B, Gibson P, Hamerlijnck D, Jarjour N, Konno S, Shen H, Vitary C, Bush A. Management of severe asthma: a European Respiratory Society/American Thoracic Society guideline. Eur Respir J. 2020;55(1):1900588.
42. Wedzicha JA Ers Co-Chair, Miravitlles M, Hurst JR, Calverley PM, Albert RK, Anzueto A, Criner GJ, Papi A, Rabe KF, Rigau D, Sliwinski P, Tonia T, Vestbo J, Wilson KC, Krishnan JA Ats Co-Chair. Management of COPD exacerbations: a European Respiratory Society/American Thoracic Society guideline. Eur Respir J. 2017;49(3):1600791.
43. https://goldcopd.org/2023-gold-report-2/
44. Han L, Ran J, Mak YW, Suen LK, Lee PH, Peiris JSM, Yang L. Smoking and influenza-associated morbidity and mortality: a systematic review and meta-analysis. Epidemiology. 2019;30:405–17.
45. Zsichla L, Müller V. Risk factors of severe COVID-19: a review of host, viral and environmental factors. Viruses. 2023;15:175.
46. Young-Wolff KC, Slama N, Alexeeff SE, Sakoda LC, Fogelberg R, Myers LC, Campbell CI, Adams AS, Prochaska JJ. Tobacco smoking and risk of SARS-CoV-2 infection and disease severity among adults in an integrated healthcare system in California. Nicotine Tob Res. 2023;25(2):211–20.

47. Benowitz NL, Goniewicz ML, Halpern-Felsher B, Krishnan-Sarin S, Ling PM, O'Connor RJ, Pentz MA, Robertson RM, Bhatnagar A. Tobacco product use and the risks of SARS-CoV-2 infection and COVID-19: current understanding and recommendations for future research. Lancet Respir Med. 2022;10:900–15.
48. Bravo-Gutiérrez OA, Falfán-Valencia R, Ramírez-Venegas A, Sansores RH, Ponciano-Rodríguez G, Pérez-Rubio G. Lung damage caused by heated tobacco products and electronic nicotine delivery systems: a systematic review. Int J Environ Res Public Health. 2021;18:4079.
49. Hayes D Jr, Board A, Calfee CS, Ellington S, Pollack LA, Kathuria H, Eakin MN, Weissman DN, Callahan SJ, Esper AM, Crotty Alexander LE, Sharma NS, Meyer NJ, Smith LS, Novosad S, Evans ME, Goodman AB, Click ES, Robinson RT, Ewart G, Twentyman E. Pulmonary and critical care considerations for e-cigarette, or vaping, product use-associated lung injury. Chest. 2022;162:256–64.
50. https://www.cdc.gov/tobacco/basic_information/e-cigarettes/severe-lung-disease.html
51. Petrache I, Gupta A, Hume PS, Rivera T, Schweitzer KS, Chu HW. Pathogenesis of E-cigarette vaping product use-associated lung injury (EVALI). Compr Physiol. 2023;13:4617–30.
52. Blount BC, Karwowski MP, Shields PG, Morel-Espinosa M, Valentin-Blasini L, Gardner M, Braselton M, Brosius CR, Caron KT, Chambers D, Corstvet J, Cowan E, De Jesús VR, Espinosa P, Fernandez C, Holder C, Kuklenyik Z, Kusovschi JD, Newman C, Reis GB, Rees J, Reese C, Silva L, Seyler T, Song MA, Sosnoff C, Spitzer CR, Tevis D, Wang L, Watson C, Wewers MD, Xia B, Heitkemper DT, Ghinai I, Layden J, Briss P, King BA, Delaney LJ, Jones CM, Baldwin GT, Patel A, Meaney-Delman D, Rose D, Krishnasamy V, Barr JR, Thomas J, Pirkle JL, Lung Injury Response Laboratory Working Group. Vitamin E acetate in bronchoalveolar-lavage fluid associated with EVALI. N Engl J Med. 2020;382:697–705.
53. Bhat TA, Kalathil SG, Bogner PN, Blount BC, Goniewicz ML, Thanavala YM. An animal model of inhaled vitamin E acetate and EVALI-like lung injury. N Engl J Med. 2020;382:1175–7.
54. Duffy B, Li L, Lu S, Durocher L, Dittmar M, Delaney-Baldwin E, Panawennage D, LeMaster D, Navarette K, Spink D. Analysis of cannabinoid-containing fluids in illicit vaping cartridges recovered from pulmonary injury patients: identification of vitamin E acetate as a major diluent. Toxics. 2020;8:8.
55. Marrocco A, Singh D, Christiani DC, Demokritou P. E-cigarette vaping associated acute lung injury (EVALI): state of science and future research needs. Crit Rev Toxicol. 2022;52:188–220.
56. Harry-Hernandez S, Thiboutot J, Wahidi MM, Giovacchini CX, De Cardenas J, Meldrum C, Los JG, Illei PB, Shojaee S, Eissenberg T, DiBardino D, Giannini H, Maldonado F, Roller L, Yarmus LB, Kapp CM. Bronchoalveolar lavage (BAL) and pathologic assessment of electronic cigarette or vaping product use-associated lung injury (EVALI): the EVALI-BAL study, a multicenter cohort. J Bronchology Interv Pulmonol. 2023;30:144–54.
57. Schekochikhina N, Meister R, Trivedi K. E-cigarette or vaping product associated lung injury (EVALI) presenting as cardiac arrest. Cureus. 2022;14:e25010.
58. Day-Lewis M, Chiel L, Gaffin J, Lee PY, Chandler MT, Son MB, Casey AM, Halyabar O. Pediatric EVALI in the age of COVID-19/MIS-C: diagnostic considerations. Hosp Pediatr. 2022;12:e249–54.
59. Aberegg SK, Cirulis MM, Maddock SD, Freeman A, Keenan LM, Pirozzi CS, Raman SM, Schroeder J, Mann H, Callahan SJ. Clinical, bronchoscopic, and imaging findings of e-cigarette, or vaping, product use-associated lung injury among patients treated at an academic medical center. JAMA Netw Open. 2020;3:e2019176.
60. Hoekstra NE, Dannull KA, Weinman JP, Liptzin DR, Hinds DM. Vaping and diffuse alveolar hemorrhage: all EVALI is not created equal. Pediatr Pulmonol. 2021;56:4057–9.
61. Cheng KA, Nichols H, McAdams HP, Henry TS, Washington L. Imaging of smoking and vaping related diffuse lung injury. Radiol Clin North Am. 2022;60:941–50.
62. Deskins SJ, Luketich SK, Al-Qatarneh S. Recurrent spontaneous pneumothorax in a 15-year-old female associated with electronic cigarettes. Pediatr Pulmonol. 2022;57:2568–70.
63. Siegel DA, Jatlaoui TC, Koumans EH, Kiernan EA, Layer M, Cates JE, Kimball A, Weissman DN, Petersen EE, Reagan-Steiner S, et al. Interim guidance for health care providers evaluat-

ing and caring for patients with suspected e-cigarette, or vaping, product use associated lung injury: United States, October 2019. MWR Morb Mortal Wkly Rep. 2019;68:919–27.
64. Rebuli ME, Rose JJ, Noël A, Croft DP, Benowitz NL, Cohen AH, Goniewicz ML, Larsen BT, Leigh N, McGraw MD, Melzer AC, Penn AL, Rahman I, Upson D, Crotty Alexander LE, Ewart G, Jaspers I, Jordt SE, Kligerman S, Loughlin CE, McConnell R, Neptune ER, Nguyen TB, Pinkerton KE, Witek TJ Jr. The E-cigarette or vaping product use-associated lung injury epidemic: pathogenesis, management, and future directions: an Official American Thoracic Society Workshop Report. Ann Am Thorac Soc. 2023;20:1–17.
65. Nemeh H, Coba V, Chulkov M, Gupta A, Yeldo N, Chamogeorgakis T, Tanaka D, Allenspach L, Simanovski J, Shanti C. Lung transplantation for the treatment of vaping-induced, irreversible, end-stage lung injury. Ann Thorac Surg. 2021;111:e353–5.
66. Blagev DP, Callahan SJ, Harris D, Collingridge DS, Hopkins RO, Eve JR, Waddoups L, Aston V, Brown S, Lanspa MJ. Prospectively assessed long-term outcomes of patients with e-cigarette- or vaping-associated lung injury. Ann Am Thorac Soc. 2022,19:1892–9.
67. Blagev DP, Harris D, Dunn AC, Guidry DW, Grissom CK, Lanspa MJ. Clinical presentation, treatment, and short-term outcomes of lung injury associated with e-cigarettes or vaping: a prospective observational cohort study. Lancet. 2019;394:2073–83.
68. Triantafyllou GA, Tiberio PJ, Zou RH, Lynch MJ, Kreit JW, McVerry BJ, Morris A, Rose JJ. Long-term outcomes of EVALI: a 1-year retrospective study. Lancet Respir Med. 2021;9:e112–3.
69. Wiens T, Taylor J, Cole C, Saravia S, Peterson J, Lunda M, Margetta J, D'Heilly P, Holzbauer S, Lynfield R. Lessons learned from the e-cigarette, or vaping, product use-associated lung injury (EVALI) outbreak response, minnesota, 2019–2020. Public Health Rep. 2022;137:1053–60.
70. Liu D, Zhu L, Yang C. The effect of preoperative smoking and smoke cessation on wound healing and infection in post-surgery subjects: a meta-analysis. Int Wound J. 2022;19:2101–6.
71. Klifto KM, Shetty PN, Slavin BR, Gurno CF, Seal SM, Asif M, Hultman CS. Impact of nicotine/smoking, alcohol, and illicit substance use on outcomes and complications of burn patients requiring hospital admission: systematic review and meta-analysis. Burns. 2020;46:1498–524.
72. Li LF, Chan RL, Lu L, Shen J, Zhang L, Wu WK, Wang L, Hu T, Li MX, Cho CH. Cigarette smoking and gastrointestinal diseases: the causal relationship and underlying molecular mechanisms. Int J Mol Med. 2014;34:372–80.
73. Berkowitz L, Schultz BM, Salazar GA, Pardo-Roa C, Sebastián VP, Álvarez-Lobos MM, Bueno SM. Impact of cigarette smoking on the gastrointestinal tract inflammation: opposing effects in Crohn's disease and ulcerative colitis. Front Immunol. 2018;9:74.
74. Xu A, Duan K, Yang W, Feng G, Wu Z, Jiang X, Li M, Liu P, Chen J. The toxic effects of electronic cigarette aerosol and cigarette smoke on cardiovascular, gastrointestinal and renal systems in mice. Sci Rep. 2023;13:12366.
75. Shapiro H, Goldenberg K, Ratiner K, Elinav E. Smoking-induced microbial dysbiosis in health and disease. Clin Sci (Lond). 2022;136:1371–87.
76. Ness-Jensen E, Lagergren J. Tobacco smoking, alcohol consumption and gastro-oesophageal reflux disease. Best Pract Res Clin Gastroenterol. 2017;31:501–8.
77. Yuan S, Chen J, Ruan X, Sun Y, Zhang K, Wang X, Li X, Gill D, Burgess S, Giovannucci E, Larsson SC. Smoking, alcohol consumption, and 24 gastrointestinal diseases: Mendelian randomization analysis. Elife. 2023;12:e84051.
78. Chen Z, Liu XA, Kenny PJ. Central and peripheral actions of nicotine that influence blood glucose homeostasis and the development of diabetes. Pharmacol Res. 2023;194:106860.
79. Durlach V, Vergès B, Al-Salameh A, Bahougne T, Benzerouk F, Berlin I, Clair C, Mansourati J, Rouland A, Thomas D, Thuillier P, Tramunt B, Le Faou AL. Smoking and diabetes interplay: a comprehensive review and joint statement. Diabetes Metab. 2022;48(6):101370.
80. Gruppen EG, Kootstra-Ros J, Kobold AM, Connelly MA, Touw D, Bos JHJ, Hak E, Links TP, Bakker SJL, Dullaart RPF. Cigarette smoking is associated with higher thyroid hormone and lower TSH levels: the PREVEND study. Endocrine. 2020;67:613–22.

81. Rehan M, Zargar UR, Sheikh IA, Alharthy SA, Almashjary MN, Abuzenadah AM, Beg MA. Potential disruption of systemic hormone transport by tobacco alkaloids using computational approaches. Toxics. 2022;10:727.
82. Abdel Fattah S, Rizk AAE, Motawie AG, Abd El-Galil TI, El Sebaie M. Effects of nicotine on rat adrenal gland: crosstalk between oxidative and inflammatory markers, and amelioration by melatonin. Biotech Histochem. 2019;94:234–43.
83. Yousaf A, Patterson J, Hobbs G, Davis SM, Yousaf M, Hafez M, Albandar H, Hogan T, Kolodney J. Smoking is associated with adrenal adenomas and adrenocortical carcinomas: a nationwide multicenter analysis. Cancer Treat Res Commun. 2020;25:100206.
84. Nagasawa Y, Yamamoto R, Rakugi H, Isaka Y. Cigarette smoking and chronic kidney diseases. Hypertens Res. 2012;35:261–5.
85. Xia J, Wang L, Ma Z, Zhong L, Wang Y, Gao Y, He L, Su X. Cigarette smoking and chronic kidney disease in the general population: a systematic review and meta-analysis of prospective cohort studies. Nephrol Dial Transplant. 2017;32:475–87.
86. Jiang S, Quan DV, Sung JH, Lee MY, Ha H. Cigarette smoke inhalation aggravates diabetic kidney injury in rats. Toxicol Res (Camb.). 2019;8:964–71.
87. Staplin N, Haynes R, Herrington WG, Reith C, Cass A, Fellström B, Jiang L, Kasiske BL, Krane V, Levin A, Walker R, Wanner C, Wheeler DC, Landray MJ, Baigent C, Emberson J, SHARP Collaborative Group. Smoking and adverse outcomes in patients With CKD: the study of heart and renal protection (SHARP). Am J Kidney Dis. 2016;68:371–80.
88. Hellemons ME, Agarwal PK, van der Bij W, Verschuuren EA, Postmus D, Erasmus ME, Navis GJ, Bakker SJ. Former smoking is a risk factor for chronic kidney disease after lung transplantation. Am J Transplant. 2011;11(11):2490–8.
89. Liu X, Peveri G, Bosetti C, Bagnardi V, Specchia C, Gallus S, Lugo A. Dose-response relationships between cigarette smoking and kidney cancer: a systematic review and meta-analysis. Crit Rev Oncol Hematol. 2019;142:86–93.
90. Xu Y, Qi Y, Zhang J, Lu Y, Song J, Dong B, Kong W, Xue W, Huang Y. The impact of smoking on survival in renal cell carcinoma: a systematic review and meta-analysis. Tumour Biol. 2014;35:6633–40.
91. Oliveira Coelho F, Andrade L. Smoking and kidney disease: risk factors, challenges, and preventive strategies. Contrib Nephrol. 2021;199:179–87.

Chapter 7
The Impact of Cannabis Use Disorder on Critical Illness

Zyad J. Carr and Eric Strand

Epidemiology

There has been a global increase in the use of cannabis and its derivatives over the past two decades, with nearly 4% of the global population reporting its use [1]. Cannabis and its derivative compounds have been studied over the past three decades for the treatment of psychiatric disorders (mood disorders, post-traumatic stress disorders), anorexia, and the induction of apoptosis in cancer cells. In the United States, this has led to a high-volume medicinal cannabinoid trade within a medical licensing framework. The abuse potential remains a controversial public and medical topic. In the United States, state-level legal frameworks have continued to relax punitive regulations regarding its use and possession, making it an increasingly accessible and socially accepted recreational drug. It remains classified as a Schedule I drug at the federal government level in the United States. Although abuse potential and physical dependence are lower in comparison to other Schedule I drugs, cannabis use disorder (CUD) is recognized and defined by the Diagnostic and Statistical Manual of Mental Disorders (DSM-IV-TR) as the pathological use of cannabis despite its perceived psychological, physical, or social impact. Approximately 9% of cannabis users experience addiction, with 20% reporting that their use began during their teenage or young adulthood.

In this evolving environment, awareness of the spectrum of cannabis use disorders is important for intensive care unit staff. Habitual users of cannabis compounds may have psychological, physical, and physiological end-organ dysfunction related to chronic cannabis use. The pathophysiological effects of acute and chronic cannabis use relevant to medical care in the ICU are discussed below.

Z. J. Carr (✉) · E. Strand
Department of Anesthesiology, Division of Critical Care Medicine, Yale University School of Medicine, New Haven, CT, USA
e-mail: zyad.carr@yale.edu; eric.Strand@yale.edu

K. Karamchandani, J. E. Grant (eds.), *Substance Use Disorders in Adult Critically Ill Patients*, https://doi.org/10.1007/978-3-031-67069-5_7

Pharmacokinetics and Pharmacodynamics

The botanical compound contains over 500 biologically active chemical compounds, complicating clinical investigations of both its positive and negative impact. Δ^9-Tetrahydrocannabinol (THC) is the primary psychoactive compound that exerts the psychiatric effects from the consumption of cannabis [2]. The absorption of cannabinoids is rapid, and peak plasma concentrations are observed after 8–10 min (inhalation), 30 min (sublingual administration), 2 h (transdermal administration), and 2 h after oral ingestion. Cannabinoids are metabolized by the liver (P450 isoenzyme family) after inhalation, absorption, or ingestion, and the plasma half-life is approximately 20–30 h. Avid tissue uptake via fat accumulation results in even longer periods of metabolite excretion up to 30 days. Δ^9-Tetrahydrocannabinol (THC) exerts its primary effects through agonistic or antagonistic actions at the cannabinoid receptor sites. Two unique G-protein-coupled cannabinoid receptors have been identified, the CB_1 and CB_2 receptors. These receptors are coupled via inhibitory G (G_i) proteins and arachidonic acid and serotonin (5-HT_3) ion channels. CB_1 receptors, of which activation produces the psychogenic and cardiovascular effects, are densely found in the brain and peripheral nervous system, as well as the peripheral organs, including the gastrointestinal tract, spleen, and heart. CB_2 receptors are predominately found among immune cells and immune tissues, including the spleen, tonsils, and a wide variety of human leukocytes. The endocannabinoids are the primary ligands for these receptors and have been identified as arachidonoylethanolamide (anandamide) and 2-archidonylglycerol (2-AG). Both appear to exert their functions as stimulus-dependent neurotransmitters or neuromodulators. Special consideration of the synthetic cannabimimetics, commonly referred to as the synthetic cannabinoids, should also be acknowledged. These compounds were originally developed to achieve high CB1 and CB2 cannabinoid receptor selectivity and high therapeutic activity. The illicit drug trade has exploited published scientific data to develop and synthesize these cannabis alternatives, which are frequently sold as herbal products, incense, or potpourri. Some synthetic cannabinoids may have fivefold the binding affinity to the cannabinoid CB1 receptor. These compounds have contributed to a dramatic increase in emergency department contacts related to cannabinoid substance-related adverse events. Toxicity symptoms include tachycardia, seizures, and hallucinations [3].

Neurological/Psychiatric

Endogenous CB1 receptor activity has been observed to exert modulatory activity on learning, memory, motor control, and sleep cycles [4]. Neurological and psychiatric manifestations are the predominant features of acute/chronic cannabis use or toxicity. Although the consequences of acute cannabis intoxication are generally mild, select patients may have significant psychological or cognitive impairments that may impact ICU care. ICU management, often for admission not directly related to cannabis use, can be negatively impacted by the presence of acute cannabis intoxication, cannabis intoxication delirium, cannabis-induced psychotic disorder, cannabis-induced sleep disorder, and acute cannabis withdrawal [5]. Cannabis intoxication is defined by the recent use of cannabis with behavioral impairment (motor coordination, impaired judgement, anxiety, or paranoia) and physiological perturbations (tachycardia). Cannabis withdrawal is associated with an elicited history of daily or near-daily use for greater than 1 month with psychological manifestations of irritability, aggression, anxiety, insomnia, and depressive symptoms. Furthermore, habitual users of cannabis have a higher incidence of underlying psychiatric disorders and associated substance use disorders, which may enhance the environment for overt delirium or psychosis after cannabis ingestion. Evidence strongly suggests that chronic cannabis use increases the risk of psychotic disorders, although longitudinal studies are needed to determine causation [6]. Anxiety, panic attacks, insomnia, and paranoia are the most commonly reported psychiatric symptoms related to acute cannabis intoxication. The most severe portion of the spectrum may result in cannabis intoxication delirium or cannabis-induced psychotic disorder. Acute cannabis-induced psychotic disorder (CIPD) presents with symptoms similar to acute psychosis, including hallucinations, delusions, paranoia, psychomotor agitation, and potentially aggressive behavior. This disorder has been induced in healthy volunteer studies exposed to THC, with behavioral symptoms nearly indistinguishable from endogenous psychosis [7]. Treatment of CIPD remains supportive, but the use of typical and atypical antipsychotic medications (olanzapine and haloperidol) has been found to provide symptom reduction [8]. Cannabis intoxication delirium (CID) presents with similar findings as ICU-related delirium but increased focus on the symptoms of inattention, awareness, and cognitive disturbances (memory deficits, visuospatial ability, or language impairment) and a close temporal relationship with cannabis use. Its presence may complicate neurological workup and assessment or mask other, more serious, neurological conditions. Cannabis-induced sleep disorder is generally characterized by a persistent impairment in sleep associated with cannabis intoxication or acute withdrawal. Similarly, its presence may enhance or contribute to ICU-related delirium, although there is no direct clinical data to support this assumption.

There has been conflicting evidence on the use of cannabis and its derivatives in the management of select neurological disorders. Cannabidiol has been found to have favorable properties in the management of treatment-resistant epilepsy [9]. Cannabis and its effects on the perception of acute and chronic pain is a topic of growing interest and controversy. A systematic review of 20 randomized placebo-controlled studies applying cannabis for the treatment of acute, chronic, or cancer pain failed to find significant chronic or postoperative pain management benefits and concluded that the psychiatric depressant effects may limit any usefulness in medical practice [10]. Similarly, Giossi and colleagues performed a meta-analysis of randomized placebo-controlled studies of cannabinoids for the treatment of chronic primary pain and found little benefit in chronic pain relief [11].

More important to ICU care, cannabis users have been observed to have high cross-tolerance to traditional sedative-hypnotics (midazolam, propofol) used for the purposes of ICU sedation [12, 13]. This cross-tolerance is particularly well understood by anesthesiology practitioners, where higher doses of propofol, hydromorphone, and higher inhalational anesthetic gas requirements have been reported in the literature [14, 15]. Higher analgesic requirements have also been reported in the literature. Studies have reported that chronic cannabis administration resulted in 23% higher opioid requirements after surgery and higher postoperative pain scores at rest and at movement [16, 17]. This may result in challenges in the management of mechanically ventilated patients, and the ICU practitioner should remain vigilant to increased sedation and analgesic requirements in chronic cannabis users requiring sedation or analgesic regimens.

Cardiovascular

THC has several actions on the cardiovascular system, which are mediated through its activation of the CB1 cannabinoid receptor. Activation of the CB1 cannabinoid receptor has been observed to modulate negative inotropy and has vasodilatory properties, generally precipitating sympathetic nervous system activation and parasympathetic suppression. Physiologically, this results in tachycardia with an increased risk of arrhythmias, endothelial dysfunction, and, when chronic, vascular smooth muscle proliferation. The effects of cannabidiol when taken alongside THC are more variable. CBD promotes both vasodilation and vasoconstriction on different vascular beds and can be implicated in both tachycardia and bradycardia events. Clinical studies have suggested that cannabis users are at higher risk for adverse cardiovascular events, but these studies may be confounded by contaminant tobacco and other drug use [18]. Similarly, there appears to be a relationship between the enhanced sympathomimetic activity associated with cannabis ingestion and cardiac arrhythmias. Increased atrial fibrillation, ventricular arrhythmias, and sudden cardiac death have been implicated with cannabis ingestion [19]. A systematic review concluded that cannabis-induced tachycardia was common (61% of Level I-III articles), with 29% of Level I-III studies reporting specific dysrhythmia such as atrial fibrillation, atrial flutter, atrioventricular blocks, and ventricular dysrhythmias [20]. For patients who arrive at the ICU after recent use, there is a possible increased risk of demand-related acute myocardial infarction. This has been postulated to be related to elevated carboxyhemoglobin levels, chronic vascular inflammation, and theorized abnormalities in the coagulation cascade. A systematic review of acute coronary syndrome in patients reporting inhaled cannabis use in 7/12 Level I-III studies found an increased risk of acute coronary syndrome and chronic cardiovascular disease in this population [21].

Pulmonary

Given the heavy particulate and volatile compounds associated with cannabis smoking/inhalation, patients may be prone to significant cannabis related pulmonary disease. Compared to tobacco, cannabis smoking results in a nearly fivefold increase in blood carboxyhemoglobin levels, a threefold increase in inhaled tar compounds, and an increased tar compound retention [22]. In addition, cannabis inhalation is known to impair airway ciliated cells responsible for the mobilization of mucus, and THC has immunosuppressive properties, which may contribute to airway health. A retrospective study examined 35,114 individuals for respiratory-related emergency room (ER) visitations and observed that cannabis users had a significantly increased risk of respiratory-related ER visit or hospitalization (OR 1.22, 95% CI 1.13–1.31) [23]. Despite this increase, cumulative marijuana use does not appear to contribute to the adverse changes in spirometry typically observed with tobacco smoking [24]. It does increase the risk of severe bronchitis at low exposure and increase airway resistance without evidence of airflow obstruction or impairment of gas exchange [25]. Mechanical ventilation may be affected by both an increase in sedation requirements related to cross-tolerance with sedative-hypnotic agents and airway hyperreactivity that may result in ventilator dyssynchrony issues [26].

Gastrointestinal

Due to its many effects on the gastrointestinal tract, cannabis has been promoted for the treatment of inflammatory bowel disease, nausea, and anorexia. While there is partial evidence to support cannabis usage in certain GI diseases, there are several GI effects that must be considered in the ICU setting. Cannabis slows gastric emptying and increases fasting gastric volume through its effect on cannabinoid receptors in the mesenteric nervous system [27]. Paradoxically, chronic cannabis smokers may experience cannabis-induced hyperemesis syndrome. This syndrome is thought to be related to the abuse of high-potency cannabinoids or via adrenocorticotropic hormone-mediated release of stored cannabinoids in adipocytes. For mild cases, the use of hot showers or capsaicin is effective in managing symptoms via stimulation of transient receptor potential vanilloid 1 (TRPV1) receptors. More severe cases may require the use of antiemetics, benzodiazepines, or anti-dopaminergic agents, such as haloperidol or droperidol [28]. There is incomplete evidence regarding the effect of cannabis on the liver. Although not directly hepatotoxic, stimulation of CB1 receptors may be associated with increased steatosis and fibrosis. Conversely, CB2 receptor stimulation has been associated with decreased rates of liver inflammation. Clinical studies have demonstrated both harm and benefit with cannabis usage in the setting of comorbid liver disease [29].

Renal

There has been limited research regarding the effects of cannabis on renal disease. To date, there is no link between cannabis usage, acute kidney injury (AKI), or the worsening of end-stage renal disease (ESRD) [30]. At least one study has demonstrated an increased risk of diabetes-related kidney disease in type 2 diabetes mellitus patients who consumed recreational cannabis [31].

Hematological

Similar to other illicit compounds, the data regarding the impact of cannabinoid compounds on the hematological system is scant. Chronic synthetic cannabinoid use has been associated with alterations in function, morphology, distribution, and index of circulating blood cells, evidence of higher levels of inflammatory cells and subclinical megaloblastic anemia with iron deficiency [32]. The findings of increased red cell indices have been previously observed to contribute to a higher risk of venous thrombosis [33]. Similarly, indirect preclinical evidence investigating endocannabinoid 2-arachidonoylglycerol (2-AG) found increased platelet aggregation and deformation, suggesting enhanced platelet aggregation [34]. Cannabinoid-positive urine tests are associated with increased hospitalization for vaso-occlusive crisis in patients harboring sickle cell disease. The authors suggested that this was not related to an underlying increase in the severity of sickle cell disease but rather as a signal of either the severity of the underlying disease (as cannabinoids were used for adjunctive pain relief) or the combined use of cannabinoids with other illicit substances, resulting in poor decision-making regarding disease management [35]. Although the etiology remains unclear, patients with cannabis use disorders have been observed to have a higher 90-day perioperative thromboembolic incidence and odds following primary total knee arthroplasty [2.79% vs. 1.78%; OR = 1.58 (95% CI 1.25–1.99) $p < 0.0001$] suggesting an aggressive approach to thromboprophylaxis in the ICU may be warranted [36].

Endocrine

The impact of cannabinoids on the endocrine system has focused on its association with fertility (male predominant; reduction in circulating plasma testosterone and sperm counts) and hormonal imbalances (polycystic ovarian syndrome); however, it appears to widely impact the endocrine system [37]. Chronic cannabinoid use does not appear to impact thyroid function but may have modulatory effects on cortisol [38]. Acute cannabis toxicity may increase cortisol secretion, but chronic cannabis users exhibit elevated basal cortisol levels and disrupted diurnal cortisol secretion, suggesting that chronic cannabis use blunts the hypothalamic-pituitary-adrenal axis [39, 40]. The implications of this hypercortisolemia in the critically ill are unclear, but practitioners should remain cautious of this phenomenon during the care of chronic cannabis users. Acute consumption of cannabis has been shown to induce glucose intolerance in pre-clinical and healthy volunteer studies. This is countered by both epidemiological studies that have found a lower prevalence of obesity and diabetes mellitus in chronic cannabis users and clinical studies that have observed increased insulin release and decreased fasting blood glucose levels in chronic cannabis use.

Infectious Disease

Little is known regarding the effect of endocannabinoids or exogenous cannabis use on the immune system's response to infection. Healthy volunteer studies have demonstrated altered monocyte phenotype and reduced tumor necrosis factor-α (TNF-α) in patients with chronic cannabis use (5 or more uses/week) [41]. Similarly, pre-clinical evidence in mice treated with cannabidiol (CBD) observed reduced systemic inflammation in a lipopolysaccharide (LPS)-induced cytokine storm model of sepsis [42]. A myriad of studies have demonstrated the anti-inflammatory activity of exogenous THC and CBD via suppression of pro-inflammatory mediators and immunomodulatory activity, but it is not fully understood if this negatively impacts the complex immunological cascade related to sepsis. Endocannabinoid signaling systems reduce inducible nitric oxide synthase (iNOS) activity, Interleukin-6 (IL-6), TNF-α, IL-1β, and inhibit neutrophil chemotaxis [43]. Clinical studies of the endocannabinoid system, namely, anandamide (AEA) and 2-AG, found that lower AEA was associated with longer hospital length of stay [OR: 23.59 (95% CI: 3.03–183.8) $p = 0.003$] in patients with confirmed sepsis [44]. A retrospective cohort analysis of perioperative outcomes after spine surgery in patients with or without the diagnosis of cannabis use disorder found similar perioperative mortality but higher rates of perioperative septicemia or sepsis [OR 1.5 (95% CI: 1.0–2.5) $p = 0.031$] and length of stay (7.1 vs. 5.2 days, $p < 0.001$) [45]. Similar perioperative findings have been demonstrated in patients with active cannabis use and perioperative complications after ruptured intracranial aneurysms, observing a higher length of stay, sepsis, and acute kidney injury [46].

Conclusion

It is important to note that cannabis remains classified as a schedule I controlled drug by the federal government. Under this classification, prospective clinical studies have been severely limited. Natural cannabis products are also heterogenous in their concentrations of various cannabinoids and terpenes, producing issues of clinical reproducibility. Numerous areas of both exogenous and endogenous cannabinoid research are needed to further characterize ICU care and management (Fig. 7.1). Supportive evidence for medicinal cannabis extracts has been demonstrated for the symptomatic treatment of subtypes of chronic pain, seizure disorders, muscle spasticity, nausea/emesis syndromes, and appetite stimulation [47, 48]. Cannabis-related negative physiological effects may directly impact ICU care and mandate an understanding of its potential negative effects. Neurological manifestations of acute cannabis complications may complicate sedation management due to sedative-hypnotic cross-tolerance, require enhanced delirium management strategies, and disrupt sleep synchrony in the ICU. Acute intoxication

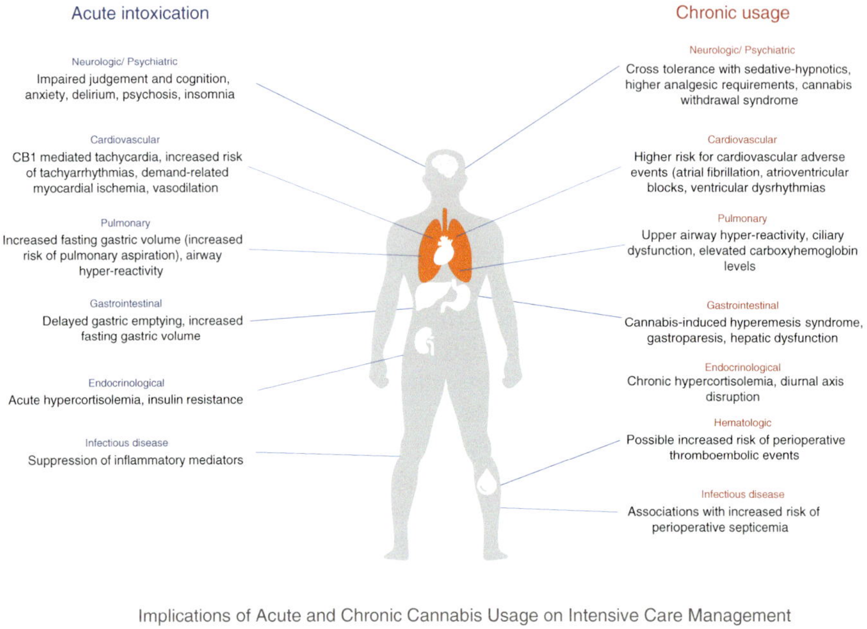

Fig. 7.1 A synopsis of acute and chronic implications of cannabis usage on intensive care management

may precipitate superimposed tachycardia and heighten the risk of tachyarrhythmias and demand-related myocardial ischemia in admitted patients. Although not proven, chronic cannabis users requiring mechanical ventilation may require aggressive pulmonary care to reduce the risk of ventilator-associated pneumonia, given its depressant effects on the immune system and ciliary activity. Hyperemesis syndromes in patients with acute cannabis use should be monitored and diagnosed to avoid distracting from other more serious primary gastrointestinal disorders. The cannabinoid's myriad downstream effects on the immune system need better characterization of its clinical relevance to ICU practitioners. Particularly concerning is the evidence regarding the increased incidence of sepsis and the increased length of stay after sepsis diagnosis. The relationship to the chronic hypercortisolemia exhibited in chronic cannabis users is unclear. Although there is no evidence of increased mortality, further characterization of cannabis-related complications during sepsis and other medical conditions is urgently required to identify mitigating strategies. Exploratory findings have suggested an increased risk of thromboembolic phenomena in chronic cannabis users, ICU practitioners should remain vigilant regarding thromboprophylaxis regarding this newly characterized problem. The relatively limited scientific knowledge and vast number of active compounds in botanical cannabis need substantial further clinical and preclinical research to determine their impact on ICU care.

References

1. Peacock A, Leung J, Larney S, Colledge S, Hickman M, Rehm J, et al. Global statistics on alcohol, tobacco and illicit drug use: 2017 status report. Addiction. 2018;113(10):1905–26.
2. Grotenhermen F. Pharmacokinetics and pharmacodynamics of cannabinoids. Clin Pharmacokinet. 2003;42(4):327–60.
3. Elsohly MA, Gul W, Wanas AS, Radwan MM. Synthetic cannabinoids: analysis and metabolites. Life Sci. 2014;97(1):78–90.
4. Zou S, Kumar U. Cannabinoid receptors and the endocannabinoid system: signaling and function in the central nervous system. Int J Mol Sci. 2018;19(3):833.
5. Patel J, Marwaha R. Cannabis use disorder. [Updated 2022 Jul 11]. StatPearls Publishing; 2023; 2022.
6. Moore THM, Zammit S, Lingford-Hughes A, Barnes TRE, Jones PB, Burke M, Lewis G. Cannabis use and risk of psychotic or affective mental health outcomes: a systematic review. Lancet (London, England). 2007;370(9584):319–28.
7. D'Souza DC, Perry E, MacDougall L, Ammerman Y, Cooper T, Wu YT, et al. The psychotomimetic effects of intravenous delta-9-tetrahydrocannabinol in healthy individuals: implications for psychosis. Neuropsychopharmacology. 2004;29(8):1558–72.
8. Crippa JA, Derenusson GN, Chagas MH, Atakan Z, Martín-Santos R, Zuardi AW, Hallak JE. Pharmacological interventions in the treatment of the acute effects of cannabis: a systematic review of literature. Harm Reduct J. 2012;9:7.
9. Devinsky O, Marsh E, Friedman D, Thiele E, Laux L, Sullivan J, et al. Cannabidiol in patients with treatment-resistant epilepsy: an open-label interventional trial. Lancet Neurol. 2016;15(3):270–8.
10. Campbell FA, Tramer MR, Carroll D, Reynolds DJ, Moore RA, McQuay HJ. Are cannabinoids an effective and safe treatment option in the management of pain? A qualitative systematic review. BMJ (Clin Res Ed). 2001;323(7303):13–6.
11. Giossi R, Carrara F, Padroni M, Bilancio MC, Mazzari M, Enisci S, et al. Systematic review and meta-analysis seem to indicate that cannabinoids for chronic primary pain treatment have limited benefit. Pain Ther. 2022;11(4):1341–58.
12. Nasser Y, Biala S, Chau M, Partridge ACR, Yang JY, Lethebe BC, et al. Baseline cannabinoid use is associated with increased sedation requirements for outpatient endoscopy. Cannabis Cannabinoid Res. 2022;95:AB50.
13. Lynn RSR, Galinkin JL. Cannabis, e-cigarettes and anesthesia. Curr Opin Anaesthesiol. 2020;33(3):318–26.
14. Davidson EM, Raz N, Eyal AM. Anesthetic considerations in medical cannabis patients. Curr Opin Anaesthesiol. 2020;33(6):832–40.
15. Holmen IC, Beach JP, Kaizer AM, Gumidyala R. The association between preoperative cannabis use and intraoperative inhaled anesthetic consumption: a retrospective study. J Clin Anesth. 2020;67:109980.
16. McLaren-Blades A, Ladha K, Goel A, Manoo V, Kotteeswaran Y, Gee YY, et al. Perioperative pain and addiction interdisciplinary network (PAIN): protocol for the perioperative management of cannabis and cannabinoid-based medicines using a modified Delphi process. BMJ Open. 2020;10(7):e036472.
17. Jamal N, Korman J, Musing M, Malavade A, Coleman BL, Siddiqui N, Friedman Z. Effects of pre-operative recreational smoked cannabis use on opioid consumption following inflammatory bowel disease surgery: a historical cohort study. Eur J Anaesthesiol. 2019;36(9):705–6.
18. Page RL 2nd, Allen LA, Kloner RA, Carriker CR, Martel C, Morris AA, et al. Medical marijuana, recreational cannabis, and cardiovascular health: a scientific statement from the American Heart Association. Circulation. 2020;142(10):e131–e52.
19. Rezkalla S, Kloner RA. Cardiovascular effects of marijuana. Trends Cardiovasc Med. 2019;29(7):403–7.

20. Richards JR, Blohm E, Toles KA, Jarman AF, Ely DF, Elder JW. The association of cannabis use and cardiac dysrhythmias: a systematic review. Clin Toxicol (Phila). 2020;58(9):861–9.
21. Richards JR, Bing ML, Moulin AK, Elder JW, Rominski RT, Summers PJ, Laurin EG. Cannabis use and acute coronary syndrome. Clin Toxicol (Phila). 2019;57(10):831–41.
22. Wu TC, Tashkin DP, Djahed B, Rose JE. Pulmonary hazards of smoking marijuana as compared with tobacco. N Engl J Med. 1988;318(6):347–51.
23. Vozoris NT, Zhu J, Ryan CM, Chow CW, To T. Cannabis use and risks of respiratory and all-cause morbidity and mortality: a population-based, data-linkage, cohort study. BMJ Open Respir Res. 2022;9(1):e001216.
24. Kempker JA, Honig EG, Martin GS. The effects of marijuana exposure on expiratory airflow. A study of adults who participated in the U.S. National Health and Nutrition Examination Study. Ann Am Thorac Soc. 2015;12(2):135–41.
25. Gracie K, Hancox RJ. Cannabis use disorder and the lungs. Addiction. 2021;116(1):182–90.
26. Flisberg P, Paech MJ, Shah T, Ledowski T, Kurowski I, Parsons R. Induction dose of propofol in patients using cannabis. Eur J Anaesthesiol. 2009;26(3):192–5.
27. Camilleri M. Cannabinoids and gastrointestinal motility: pharmacology, clinical effects, and potential therapeutics in humans. Neurogastroenterol Motil. 2018;30(9):e13370.
28. Perisetti A, Gajendran M, Dasari CS, Bansal P, Aziz M, Inamdar S, et al. Cannabis hyperemesis syndrome: an update on the pathophysiology and management. Ann Gastroenterol. 2020;33(6):571–8.
29. Cohen L, Neuman MG. Cannabis and the gastrointestinal tract. J Pharm Pharm Sci. 2020;23:301–13.
30. Potukuchi PK, Moradi H, Park F, Kaplan C, Thomas F, Dashputre AA, et al. Cannabis use and risk of acute kidney injury in patients with advanced chronic kidney disease transitioning to dialysis. Cannabis Cannabinoid Res. 2023;8(1):138–47.
31. Porr CJ, Rios P, Bajaj HS, Egan AM, Huot C, Batten R, et al. The effects of recreational cannabis use on glycemic outcomes and self-management behaviours in people with type 1 and type 2 diabetes: a rapid review. Syst Rev. 2020;9(1):187.
32. Guzel D, Yazici AB, Yazici E, Erol A. Alterations of the hematologic cells in synthetic cannabinoid users. J Clin Lab Anal. 2017;31(6):e22131.
33. Rezende SM, Lijfering WM, Rosendaal FR, Cannegieter SC. Hematologic variables and venous thrombosis: red cell distribution width and blood monocyte count are associated with an increased risk. Haematologica. 2014;99(1):194–200.
34. Baldassarri S, Bertoni A, Bagarotti A, Sarasso C, Zanfa M, Catani MV, et al. The endocannabinoid 2-arachidonoylglycerol activates human platelets through non-CB1/CB2 receptors. J Thromb Haemost. 2008;6(10):1772–9.
35. Ballas SK. The use of cannabis by patients with sickle cell disease increased the frequency of hospitalization due to vaso-occlusive crises. Cannabis Cannabinoid Res. 2017;2(1):197–201.
36. Vakharia RM, Sodhi N, Anis HK, Ehiorobo JO, Mont MA, Roche MW. Patients who have cannabis use disorder have higher rates of venous thromboemboli, readmission rates, and costs following primary total knee arthroplasty. J Arthroplast. 2020;35(4):997–1002.
37. Meah F, Lundholm M, Emanuele N, Amjed H, Poku C, Agrawal L, Emanuele MA. The effects of cannabis and cannabinoids on the endocrine system. Rev Endocr Metab Disord. 2022;23(3):401–20.
38. Bonnet U. Chronic cannabis abuse, delta-9-tetrahydrocannabinol and thyroid function. Pharmacopsychiatry. 2013;46(1):35–6.
39. van Leeuwen AP, Creemers HE, Greaves-Lord K, Verhulst FC, Ormel J, Huizink AC. Hypothalamic-pituitary-adrenal axis reactivity to social stress and adolescent cannabis use: the TRAILS study. Addiction. 2011;106(8):1484–92.
40. Ranganathan M, Braley G, Pittman B, Cooper T, Perry E, Krystal J, D'Souza DC. The effects of cannabinoids on serum cortisol and prolactin in humans. Psychopharmacology (Berl). 2009;203(4):737–44.
41. Lisano JK, Kisiolek J, Flores V, Smoak P, Pullen NA, Stewart LK. Chronic cannabis use is associated with altered monocyte phenotype, immune response, and depression in physically active individuals. Can J Physiol Pharmacol. 2023;101(6):316–26.

42. Maayah ZH, Ferdaoussi M, Alam A, Takahara S, Silver H, Soni S, et al. Cannabidiol suppresses cytokine storm and protects against cardiac and renal injury associated with sepsis. Cannabis Cannabinoid Res. 2022.
43. Dinu AR, Rogobete AF, Bratu T, Popovici SE, Bedreag OH, Papurica M, et al. Cannabis sativa revisited-crosstalk between microRNA expression, inflammation, oxidative stress, and endocannabinoid response system in critically ill patients with sepsis. Cells. 2020;9(2):307.
44. Šahinović I, Mandić S, Mihić D, Duvnjak M, Loinjak D, Sabadi D, et al. Endocannabinoids, anandamide and 2-arachidonoylglycerol, as prognostic markers of sepsis outcome and complications. Cannabis Cannabinoid Res. 2022;8:802.
45. Chiu RG, Patel S, Siddiqui N, Nunna RS, Mehta AI. Cannabis abuse and perioperative complications following inpatient spine surgery in the United States. Spine (Phila Pa 1976). 2021;46(11):734–43.
46. Chiu RG, Fuentes AM, Patil SN, Chiu R, McGuire LS, Mehta AI. Cannabis abuse and perioperative complications after treatment of intracranial aneurysms: a nationwide analysis. World Neurosurg. 2022;158:e184–e95.
47. Legare CA, Raup-Konsavage WM, Vrana KE. Therapeutic potential of cannabis, cannabidiol, and cannabinoid-based pharmaceuticals. Pharmacology. 2022;107(3–4):131–49.
48. Whiting PF, Wolff RF, Deshpande S, Di Nisio M, Duffy S, Hernandez AV, et al. Cannabinoids for medical use: a systematic review and meta-analysis. JAMA. 2015;313(24):2456–73.

Chapter 8
Stimulant Use Disorder

Kristin Reinaker and Jami Johnson

Abbreviations

ACC:	American College of Cardiology
AHA:	American Heart Association
AKI:	Acute kidney injury
BB:	Beta blocker(s)
CAACS:	Cocaine-associated acute coronary syndrome
CNS:	Central nervous system
ECG:	Electrocardiogram
EF:	Ejection fraction
GDMT:	Goal-directed medical therapy
HF:	Heart failure
ICD:	Implantable cardioverter defibrillator(s)
IM:	Intramuscular
Kg:	Kilogram
LVAD:	Left ventricular assist device(s)
MDA:	3,4-methylenedioxyamphetamine
MDE:	3,4-methylenedioxy-N-ethylamphetamine
MDMA:	3,4-methelenedioxymethamphetamine
Ng:	Milligram
MI:	Myocardial infarction

K. Reinaker (✉)
Department of Pharmacy Practice and Administration, Ernest Mario School of Pharmacy, Rutgers, The State University of New Jersey, Ewing, NJ, USA
e-mail: kbohnenberger@pharmacy.rutgers.edu

J. Johnson
Oklahoma Center for Poison and Drug Information, University of Oklahoma College of Pharmacy, Oklahoma City, OK, USA

K. Karamchandani, J. E. Grant (eds.), *Substance Use Disorders in Adult Critically Ill Patients*, https://doi.org/10.1007/978-3-031-67069-5_8

NSDUH: National Survey on Drug Use and Health
NSTE-ACS: Non-ST segment elevation acute coronary syndromes
PVCs: Premature ventricular contractions
SC: Synthetic cathinones
US: United States
VF: Ventricular fibrillation
VT: Ventricular tachycardia

Epidemiology

The use of stimulants, such as cocaine and amphetamines, accounts for numerous emergency department visits each year [1]. In recent years, increased rates of emergency department visits, hospitalizations, and deaths from stimulant overdose have been reported [1, 2]. According to the National Survey on Drug Use and Health (NSDUH), cocaine was used by 4.8 million people over the age of 12 in the United States (US) in 2021 [3]. Globally, the World Drug Report 2020 reported that cocaine was used by 21.5 million people in the preceding year [4]. Amphetamine use in North America was notably higher than that of the global prevalence (3.9% vs. 0.7%) in 2020, with amphetamine and "ecstasy-type" substances reportedly used in 34 million people and 20 million people aged 15–64 years, respectively [4]. In the US, methamphetamine was used by 2.5 million people (1% of the population) over the age of 12 in 2021 [3]. Furthermore, deaths in the US attributed to methamphetamine increased from several hundred per year in the 1990s to over 32,000 in 2021 [5].

History

Cocaine

Cocaine is an alkaloid contained within the leaves of the coca plant (*Erythroxylon coca*), a bush which grows extensively in Columbia, Peru, and the Plurinational State of Bolivia [4, 6]. Thought to be a gift from the royal son god Manco Cepac, leaves were mixed with lime and chewed in traditional Incan religious ceremonies as early as the sixth century [6, 7]. Additionally, native South Americans discovered that chewing coca leaves alleviated fatigue and altitude sickness, thus establishing the plant within social practices as well [7]. Following the introduction of the leaves to Europe by explorers, the alkaloid cocaine was isolated, purified, and named in 1860 [6, 7]. Thereafter, cocaine's stimulant and anesthetic properties led to its role as a pharmaceutical tool. In 1883, it was used to alleviate fatigue in Bavarian soldiers [6]. In 1884, after experimenting with its use to alleviate his own depression, Sigmund Freud proposed that cocaine be used as a stimulant, aphrodisiac, local anesthetic, and to manage asthma, digestive disorders, cachexia, and alcohol and morphine dependence [6]. The successful use of cocaine as a local anesthetic during ocular surgery and as a regional nerve block cemented its use in modern medicine in the same year [6]. Shortly thereafter, cocaine from the coca leaf and caffeine from the kola nut were incorporated into an elixir and marketed as Coca-Cola™ to become one of the most popular elixirs in the US [6, 7]. It wasn't until 1906 that the company agreed to use decocainized leaves in its formula [6]. With its incorporation into numerous products, the widespread use of cocaine made the penchant for addiction apparent. The Pure Food and Drug Act helped curtail its use when it required the disclosure of all constituents on medication labels [7]. Eight years later, in 1914, recreational use of cocaine was made illegal with the passage of the Harrison Narcotics Act, which limited the use of cocaine to medical use for local anesthesia of the mucus membranes of the nasal, oral, or laryngeal cavities [7]. This placed cocaine under strict control and subjected its use to similar penalties as opium, morphine, and heroin [6].

Despite its legal limitation to medical use, the illicit use of cocaine remains prevalent [3, 4]. Following an increase in amphetamine-related deaths in the 1960s and early 1970s, the use of cocaine rose sharply due to its role as a substitutive psychostimulant [7]. Intravenous cocaine rose in popularity as users sought to substitute injectable amphetamines. The advent of freebase and crack formulations in the late 1970s afforded new options which provided users with a similar "rush" as would be achieved with the intravenous formulation [8]. Given the propensity of rapid plasma elevations to result in addiction, it was predicted that these reports of cardiovascular toxicity would surmount [9]. As predicted, the first case of cocaine-associated myocardial infarction (MI) in the US was reported in 1982, followed by similar reports in the years that followed [10]. Recreational use of cocaine remains a major issue. Cultivation of coca reached a record high in 2021, climbing 35% from the previous year, demonstrating the sharpest year-to-year increase since 2016 [11]. The increase in supply is in response to a steep growth in demand, with the world's largest consumer market for cocaine being North America, followed by Europe [4].

Amphetamines

Amphetamine was first synthesized by G.A. Alles in 1927 while researching economic alternatives to ephedrine [12]. Like many other substances of abuse, amphetamine use began medicinally, with mixed success, for ailments ranging from morphine addiction and myasthenia gravis to seasickness and night blindness in the 1930s and into the 1940s. During this time, amphetamines were concomitantly supplied in substantial quantities to soldiers during World War II to enhance alertness and combat fatigue, with 72 million Benzedrine tablets distributed to British soldiers alone [13]. This led to more widespread recreational use of amphetamines in the 1950s and 1960s, when growing concerns over addiction led to increased regulation [12]. While the legitimate use of amphetamines declined in the 1970s and 1980s, their illicit use, especially methamphetamine, began to drastically rise. In recent decades, illicit use of amphetamines has remained a challenge, and amphetamines are the most consumed illicit substance in the world, second only to cannabis [12, 14].

Synthetic Cathinones

More recently, synthetic stimulants (Table 8.1) have emerged as cheaper alternatives to classic stimulants [15]. Often marketed as "bath salts" or "molly," synthetic cathinones (SC) are structurally related to cathinone [16]. Considered a natural amphetamine, cathinone (2-amino-1-phenylproan-1-one) is a naturally occurring alkaloid found in the khat plant (*Catha edulis*) that elicits similar stimulative effects as amphetamines [17]. Because routine methods of detecting SCs within biological samples have only recently emerged and are limited in the substances they can detect, the ability for SC use to remain undetected likely contributes to their appeal [4, 18]. Identification of all substances present in a sample is limited to costly and often inaccessible laboratory methods such as gas and liquid chromatography or high-resolution mass spectrometry [19]. Thus, despite the first SC, ephedrone (2-[methylamino]-1-phenyl-propan-1-one), being synthesized in 1928, stimulants accounted for 25% of new psychoactive substances reported globally in 2020 and 30% of newly discovered psychoactive substances detected in the US between 2018–2022 [4, 20, 21]. Following their production in China and other Asian countries, these substances enter the global market without prior pharmacologic or toxicologic testing [22]. Several reports of intoxication and fatality with SCs have been

Table 8.1 Synthetic cathinones

Group	Examples	Street names
I	Ephedrone; mephedrone; 3-methylmethcathinone; 4-ethylmethcathinone; buphedrone; pentadrone; 4-methylpentedrone; 4-methyl-N-ethylpentedrone; N-propyl pentedrone; 4-chloropentedrone; n-ethylhexedrone; mexedrone; brephedrone; clephedrone; flephedrone; 3-fluoromethcathinone; ethcathinone; 4-chloroethcathinone; 4-MEC; methedrone; N,N-dimethylcathinone; 2,3-dimethylmethcathinine; 2,4-dimethylmethcathinone; 3,4-dimethylmethcathinone	m-cat, meph, drone, miaow, crank, gagers, go-fast, goob, qat, the C, Cadillac express, bathtub speed, wonder star, wild cat, jeff, mulka, 4-MMC, meow meow, bounce, mad cow
II	Methylone, dimethylone, ethylone, butylone, dibutylone, pentylone, dipentylone, N-ethylpentylone	explosion, bubbles, MDMCAT, ease, m11, bk-MDEA, MDEC
III	Pyrovalerone, α -PVP, 4-F-PVP, 4-Cl-PVP, 4-MeO-PVP, α-PPP, 4-Me-PPP, 4-Cl-PPP, α -PBP, α -PHP, 4-F-PHP, 4-Me-PHP, PV8	flakka, gravel
IV	MDPV, MDPPP, MDPBP, MDPHP	blizzard, ivory wave, vanilla sky, energy-1, plant fertilizer, peevee
Other	Naphyrone, TH-PVP, α -PVT	bath salts, research chemicals

published, suggesting that these novel substances pose similar health risks to classic stimulants [22]. Despite evidence of these risks, few have been classified as controlled substances in the US [16].

Acute Intoxication

Cocaine

Cocaine increases the release of, inhibits the reuptake of, and sensitizes postsynaptic receptors to the catecholamines dopamine, norepinephrine, and epinephrine [23–25]. The impact of these effects on the cardiovascular system is multifaceted and includes increased myocardial oxygen demand secondary to hypertension and tachycardia, decreased coronary blood flow from vasoconstriction and vasospasm, enhanced atherogenesis, and hypercoagulability due to enhanced platelet aggregation and impaired thrombolysis [26, 27]. Furthermore, chronic exposure to high catecholamine concentrations leads to direct myocyte death and fibrosis, which reduces systolic function and increases the risk of MI, heart failure (HF), cardiomyopathy, aortic dissection, and arrhythmias [28]. Cocaine also has proarrhythmic effects due to its blockade of voltage-dependent sodium, potassium, and calcium channels, resulting in QRS and QT interval prolongation [29]. Interestingly, bradyarrhythmias including second-degree AV block with acute use and sinus bradycardia with chronic use have been reported; the mechanism behind AV block with acute use has not been confirmed in humans, but desensitization of beta receptors from repeated cocaine exposure is thought to explain the sinus bradycardia reported with chronic cocaine use [30, 31]. When smoked, cocaine produces bronchospasm, which may result from cocaine's direct effect on the airway, inhaled contaminants, thermal injury, or a pyrolytic metabolite [32, 33]. Lastly, cocaine also increases excitatory amino acid concentrations in the brain, resulting in CNS excitation, increased neuronal firing, further reuptake blockade, and an exaggerated sympathetic response [34].

Cocaine can be injected intravenously, smoked, nasally insufflated, or taken orally. The inhaled and smoked routes share similar kinetics, with the quickest onset (<1 minute) but shortest duration of action (30–60 minutes), thus contributing to its addictive potential [35]. Owing to vasoconstriction in the mucus membranes, nasal insufflation and oral administration have comparatively slower rates of absorption (1–5 minutes and 30–60 minutes, respectively) and longer durations of action (60–120 minutes and 30–140 minutes, respectively) [35, 36]. Metabolism is complex and results in both active and inactive metabolites (norcocaine, benzoylecgonine, and ecgonine methyl ester) [37]. When combined with ethanol, an active metabolite, cocaethylene, is produced, which has a longer duration of action and similar neuro- and cardiotoxic effects to cocaine, thereby prolonging its toxicity [38]. Smoking cocaine produces unique metabolites (methylecgonide and ecgonide) [39].

Acute cocaine toxicity is best described as sympathetic overactivity. Vital sign abnormalities include hypertension, tachycardia, tachypnea, and hyperthermia, with hyperthermia being the most critical [33, 40]. Other characteristic markers of sympathomimetic toxicity include mydriasis, diaphoresis, agitation, and tremors [41]. CNS manifestations of acute cocaine toxicity include headache, intracranial hemorrhage, vasospastic infarction, transient ischemic attack, coma, and seizures [42–44]. Seizures typically occur within minutes of use but have been reported up to 24 hours later [45]. Neuropsychiatric effects are dose-dependent, with low doses eliciting the desired effects of cocaine, such as euphoria and hypersexual behavior. Higher doses, however, result in agitated delirium, aggression, and hallucinations, which may cause patients to seek care [46, 47]. Acute dystonia or choreoathetoid movements, known as "crack dancing," may result from dopamine dysregulation [48]. Vasospasm of retinal vasculature can result in unilateral and bilateral vision loss [49, 50]. Ischemic colitis, intestinal infarction, and renal infarctions result from vasospasm in the gastrointestinal system [51–53]. The manifestation of vomiting or distension, suggesting bowel obstruction, should prompt an investigation for potential package concealment (e.g., body packing or stuffing). Repeated ischemic injury following nasal insufflation can result in nasal septum perforation and wound botulism [54, 55]. Rhabdomyolysis in the absence of psychomotor agitation is possible [56]. Because the anesthetizing and euphoric effects of cocaine may mask signs of traumatic injury, occult fractures should be ruled out [57]. Vasospasm, enhanced atherogenesis, and prothrombotic effects could result in limb ischemia [58, 59]. Hypoglycemia secondary to catecholamine discharge is also possible [60]. Cardiovascular manifestations include arrhythmias such as sinus tachycardia, supraventricular tachycardia, frequent premature ventricular contractions (PVCs), ventricular tachycardia (VT)/fibrillation (VF), and torsade de pointes; aortic dissection; endocarditis; chest pain; and cocaine-associated acute coronary syndrome (CAACS) [61–63]. The risk of CAACS is increased 24-fold in the 60 minutes following cocaine use, and users have a higher overall incidence of MI compared to nonusers [64]. Sudden cardiac death has also been reported in young, otherwise healthy patients [63].

Smoking cocaine results in its own symptomology. Madarosis, or the loss of eyebrow and eyelash hair, has been reported following thermal injuries from smoking cocaine [65]. Thermal injury to the airway from smoking cocaine has resulted in angioedema and oropharyngeal burns as distally as the esophagus [66, 67]. Bearing down against a closed epiglottis following nasal insufflation or smoking increases intrathoracic pressure and can result in a pneumothorax, pneumomediastinum, or pneumopericardium [68]. The term "crack lung" is used to describe the fever, hemoptysis, hypoxia, acute respiratory distress syndrome, and respiratory failure that can result from inhalational use [68]. Pulmonary infarction from vasospasm and subsequent thrombosis of the pulmonary artery has also been reported [68].

The management of acute stimulant toxicity is centered on supportive care and begins with an assessment of the patient's airway, breathing, and circulation. Should intubation be required, succinylcholine should be avoided in the cocaine-toxic patient for two reasons. First, both cocaine and succinylcholine are metabolized by plasma cholinesterase, so simultaneous exposure could prolong the toxic effects of cocaine, the paralytic effects of succinylcholine, or both [69]. Additionally, succinylcholine will increase serum potassium; its use can exacerbate hyperkalemia in patients with rhabdomyolysis, thereby increasing the risk of arrhythmias [70]. Intravenous fluids should be initiated for hypotension, volume depletion from excessive fluid losses, and rhabdomyolysis. Core body temperature should be assessed, even in a severely agitated patient, and ice water immersion should be initiated if the patient is hyperthermic [71]. Antipyretics, medications to prevent shivering (e.g., chlorpromazine, meperidine), and dantrolene are not recommended to facilitate rapid cooling as they are either ineffective or detrimental (e.g., serotonin toxicity with meperidine, seizures with chlorpromazine) [71, 72].

Agitation should be initially managed with benzodiazepines [73]. The optimal benzodiazepine is not well studied, however. Parenteral benzodiazepines with a rapid onset and peak of action, such as midazolam or diazepam, may be preferred over lorazepam, lending to easier titration and the avoidance of oversedation from repeat doses. Larger doses may be required due to cocaine-induced alterations in benzodiazepine receptor function [34]. Antipsychotics can be used, but in the setting of cocaine-induced agitation, benzodiazepines have been shown to reduce mortality to a greater extent [73]. The use of phenothiazines (e.g., chlorpromazine, prochlorperazine, fluphenazine, thioridazine) and butyrophenones (e.g., haloperidol, droperidol) as monotherapy is contraindicated in cocaine-induced agitation for reasons that include enhanced toxicity, reduced heat dissipation, worsened tachycardia, QT prolongation, and enhanced dystonia [34, 73]. Thus, if further sedation is required, rapid acting barbiturates or propofol serve as reasonable alternatives.

Benzodiazepines also serve as an effective first-line therapy for patients presenting with symptoms of cocaine-induced cardiotoxicity such as hypertension, arrhythmias, and tachycardia [74]. Nitroglycerin can be used if patients remain hemodynamically unstable despite benzodiazepines, particularly for continued chest pain and hypertension [74]. Other medications such as calcium channel blockers (nicardipine, verapamil), antiplatelets (aspirin, clopidogrel, and glycoprotein IIb/IIIa inhibitors), anticoagulants (heparin), and morphine have also been used successfully [74]. Dexmedetomidine has also been shown to mitigate tachycardia and hypertension with mixed results [75]. Phentolamine, an alpha-adrenergic antagonist, has been used with success in the setting of CAACS when given in 1 mg aliquots at 5-minute intervals [76].

Beta-blocker therapy (BBT) in patients with cocaine-induced chest pain and arrhythmias is controversial. The genesis of this controversy was data from experimental studies and reports of severe hypertension, coronary vasospasm, and death following beta blockers (BBs) use in cocaine users [64]. Unopposed alpha receptor stimulation and resultant enhanced vasoconstriction were hypothesized to explain the worsened cocaine-related cardiovascular effects observed [77]. More recent research, however, suggests that this phenomenon may be unrelated to BBT [78]. Additionally, new data suggest no difference in outcomes in active cocaine users given BB for cocaine-associated hypertension, chest pain, or tachycardia compared to non-users [79]. Current guidelines from the American Heart Association (AHA)/American College of Cardiology (ACC) suggest that treatment for patients presenting with cocaine- or methamphetamine-related non-ST segment elevation acute coronary syndromes (NSTE-ACS) should not differ from those with NSTE-ACS unrelated to cocaine or methamphetamine use unless patients demonstrate signs of active intoxication (e.g., tachycardia, hypertension) [80]. In that situation, they recommend the use of nitroglycerin with or without benzodiazepines in combination with BBT.

Sodium channel blockade is thought to be responsible for many of the wide-complex arrhythmias that occur immediately following cocaine use [81]. Because the inhibition of sodium conduction is worsened at increased heart rates and blockade increases at lower pH, sodium bicarbonate may facilitate improved conduction via both sodium loading and ameliorating acidosis [81]. The successful use of sodium bicarbonate to treat cocaine-associated wide-complex dysrhythmias and asystolic arrests has been reported [81]. Its use in managing wide-complex arrhythmias is supported in multiple statements from the AHA [82, 83]. The use of lidocaine, an antiarrhythmic that also functions to block sodium channels, in the acute setting, however, is controversial. While lidocaine reduced the seizure threshold in an animal model, no seizures were reported when lidocaine was used in a study of cocaine-associated MI in humans [81]. On the other hand, persistent or recurrent ventricular arrhythmias occurring several hours after the last use of cocaine are more likely to result from ischemia, so the use of lidocaine is reasonable [83]. The safety and efficacy of amiodarone, while common in the management of wide-complex tachycardia and refractory VT/VF, have not been evaluated in cocaine-induced arrhythmias in humans [81]. Due to its blockade of beta-adrenergic receptors, amiodarone use would theoretically share similar safety concerns to BBs.

Amphetamines

Phenylethylamines (including amphetamine and methamphetamine) are synthetic CNS stimulants that increase the activity of neurotransmitters, primarily dopamine, norepinephrine, and serotonin [84]. The activity of individual amphetamines on the various neurotransmitters depends upon chemical structure modifications that lend toward more stimulant, hallucinogenic, or empathogenic effects [85]. These structural considerations can affect the acute toxicity of the drug. However, most patients will present with general findings consistent with the sympathomimetic toxidrome, similar to acute cocaine intoxication. Special considerations for various amphetamines will be discussed below.

Amphetamines can be absorbed via a variety of routes: oral, intranasal, inhalational, rectal, and intravenous [84]. They are rapidly absorbed with bioavailability as high as 90%, depending on the route of administration and style. For example, depending upon the method of inhalation, the bioavailability of methamphetamine following smoking can range from 67% to 90% [86]. Immediately following inhalation or intravenous injection, the onset of activity is almost immediate, while taking up to 5 minutes following insufflation and up to 20 minutes after oral ingestion [87]. The duration of the activity is approximately 12 hours. Methamphetamine is metabolized primarily by the liver, but metabolites are unlikely to contribute to the clinical effects, and metabolism does not appear to be altered by chronic exposure [86]. A need to escalate dosing is more reasonably explained by a pharmacodynamic tolerance (a diminished clinical effect) than a pharmacokinetic tolerance. Acute tachyphylaxis to the subjective effects sought by users may diminish in as little as four hours, while other cardiovascular and CNS effects continue for longer (approximately 12 hours), contributing to the toxicity seen in these organ systems [88].

The symptoms of acute amphetamine intoxication are consistent with the sympathomimetic toxidrome [89]. CNS manifestations include mydriasis, agitation, anxiety, hallucinations, paranoia, seizures, suicidal ideation, confusion, psychosis, tachypnea, diaphoresis, and hyperthermia [86]. Hyperthermia not only results from increased psychomotor and metabolic activity but also decreased heat dissipation due to profound vasoconstriction [84]. Cardiovascular manifestations include hypertension, tachycardia, dysrhythmias, and vascular complications such as myocardial ischemia [90]. Dysrhythmias may range from PVCs to malignant ventricular dysrhythmias, such as VT or VF [84]. In one review, 9% of patients reported chest pain with no ECG changes [89]. Reports of conduction abnormalities such as prolonged QT intervals and subsequent polymorphic ventricular tachycardia have been reported [91]. Other reported vascular complications include intracerebral hemorrhage, cerebral infarct, MI, aortic dissection, and ischemic colitis [92–95]. Additionally, patients may experience metabolic acidosis, acute kidney injury, acute tubular necrosis, and rhabdomyolysis secondary to uncontrolled agitation and hyperthermia [89, 96–98]. These may progress to multiorgan failure and death without prompt intervention.

Several studies suggest that many methamphetamine-related fatalities are due to trauma. In a retrospective study of 7,844 emergency department (ED) visits, blunt trauma was present in 20% of patients; therefore, additional diagnostic work-up should be completed accordingly [99]. In addition to trauma, suicide and homicide are also seen, suggesting that severe psychological pathology contributes to the outcomes in these patients [100].

There is no specific antidote to treat patients with amphetamine toxicity. Acute resuscitation should lend special attention to rapid cooling, abatement of seizures, and rapid control of agitation to prevent worsened hyperthermia and rhabdomyolysis [84]. Chemical sedation is the first integral step because it works to accomplish all three while facilitating continued patient work-up. Benzodiazepines are considered excellent chemical sedation candidates for patients with acute amphetamine intoxication due to their antiepileptic activity as well as their acceptable safety profile and predictable pharmacokinetics [84]. Intravenous benzodiazepines should be administered as soon as possible; if intravenous access cannot immediately be established, then intramuscular delivery can be considered until definitive intravenous access is established. Sedation should be titrated until the patient is calm, and large doses may be required initially to reach this endpoint. Doses exceeding 100 mg of diazepam or equivalent have been reported [84].

Antipsychotics are also recommended as adjunct therapy for the management of delirium and agitation in this patient population. Haloperidol, droperidol, and olanzapine have all been studied and may be utilized depending upon the clinical situation. In a prospective, randomized study of violently agitated patients requiring chemical sedation (72% were methamphetamine toxicity), droperidol provided more rapid and greater sedation than lorazepam at the provided doses: lorazepam 2 mg (< 50 kg) or 4 mg (> 50 kg); droperidol 2.5 mg (< 50 kg) or 5 mg (> 50 kg) [101].

Ketamine has also been studied for rapid sedation in severely agitated patients. In one randomized, controlled clinical trial comparing the rapidity of onset, level of sedation, and adverse effect profile of ketamine (5 mg/kg IM) compared to midazolam (5 mg IM) plus haloperidol (5 mg IM), the authors concluded that IM ketamine provided a shorter time to adequate sedation [102].

In addition to chemical sedation, rapid cooling is instrumental in management. External cooling should be implemented [71]. Ice water immersion has been proven to cool at rates exceeding evaporative cooling. Evaporative techniques are recommended if ice-water immersion is not possible. Evidence for the use of dantrolene to facilitate cooling and muscle relaxation in this patient population is limited, though anecdotal reports of its effectiveness in 3,4-methelenedioxymethamphetami ne (MDMA) ingestion have been reported [103].

Additional supportive measures for rhabdomyolysis (intravenous fluid hydration to assure urine output targets per institutional protocol) should be implemented [104]. There is no consensus on the best fluid composition to administer, and there is no evidence to support the use of mannitol or urinary alkalinization [104].

Hemodialysis can be utilized as clinically indicated for patients with acute kidney injury, refractory acidosis, or profound electrolyte disturbances as a supportive measure, but it will not aid in the elimination of amphetamines [84].

Three methylenedioxy analogues of amphetamine are illicit recreational drugs with some distinct pharmacologic activity and are often referred to as "entactogens." The primary analogue used recreationally in the US is MDMA, colloquially referred to as "ecstasy," with others such as 3,4-methylenedioxyamphetamine (MDA, "love") and 3,4-methylenedioxy-N-ethylamphetamine (MDE, "eve") may also be encountered [105]. These analogues have similar central and peripheral effects in humans, but variable potency (with MDA being the most potent), onset (approximately 30 minutes for all, but up to 60 minutes for MDA), and duration of action (MDA 8 hours, MDMA 6 hours, MDE 3–4 hours) [106]. The primary distinguishing factor in the management of methylenedioxy analogues of amphetamines versus traditional amphetamines is the increased incidence of hyponatremia and potential for cerebral edema, as well as serotonin toxicity. MDMA has diminished CNS stimulant effects compared to other amphetamines [107]. MDMA's hyponatremic effects are well characterized and described as dilutional in nature, as an increase in water intake is linked directly to MDMA consumption, which is at least partially linked to hyperpyrexia, dry mouth, and increased thirst [107]. Additionally, MDMA increases the release of vasopressin, contributing to the development of hyponatremia [84, 107].

Withdrawal

Cocaine

Abrupt cessation of cocaine is not associated with a withdrawal syndrome. Reduced levels of consciousness, however, can occur following its binge use. Decreased consciousness ranges from lethargy and hypersomnolence to coma, and patients have trouble initiating and sustaining movement [108, 109]. Despite an inability to speak or respond to simple commands in the absence of external stimuli, neurologic and metabolic work-up is typically unrevealing [108]. Following observation, patients return to their baseline mental status 6–18 hours later [109]. The term "cocaine washed out syndrome" was coined to describe this phenomenon, and it is proposed to result from the overstimulation of the CNS followed by the subsequent depletion of neurotransmitters such as dopamine [108, 109]. Animal models of acute cocaine use support this theory, as brain levels of dopamine, norepinephrine, and serotonin increased immediately following cocaine exposure but gradually reduced until the eventual depletion was well below baseline [109]. This syndrome may mask delayed symptoms of cocaine intoxication, such as myocardial ischemia manifesting with ST elevation, within the first two weeks of cocaine abstinence [109]. The mechanism for these delayed symptoms has not been fully elucidated but is ostensibly related to a lowered threshold for vasospasm (from dopamine depletion or increased sensitivity to alpha adrenergic receptor stimulation) or a lower threshold for thrombogenesis due to enhanced platelet aggregability [34].

Amphetamines

Patients with acute amphetamine intoxication are at obvious risk for withdrawal during their hospital stay. The potential for withdrawal to develop in those with stimulant use disorder, not presenting for acute intoxication, who are admitted for other etiologies should also be anticipated, however [110]. While withdrawal symptoms are protracted, extremely uncomfortable, and may worsen a patient's condition during their stay, they are rarely life-threatening. Symptom severity depends upon a variety of factors, including length of stimulant use, dose of amphetamine typically administered, frequency of use, method of administration (for example, patients with a history of intravenous methamphetamine abuse typically have prolonged, difficult, and intense withdrawal syndromes), and presence of polysubstance abuse [111, 112]. Symptoms include fatigue, increased appetite, agitation, anxiety, insomnia, disturbed sleep, vivid and unpleasant dreams, paranoia, hallucinations, confusion, tremor, suicidal ideation, depression, craving, cognitive impairment, excessive sweating, fever, nausea, and abdominal pain [113]. The time course of withdrawal will vary, but the acute phase typically begins within 24 hours of abstinence, peaks within the first week, and lasts between 2–4 weeks [113]. The psychological symptoms (a protracted extinction phase) associated with amphetamine withdrawal may last much longer, months to years, and may be sufficiently severe as to cause relapse. Withdrawal symptoms should be assessed utilizing the Amphetamine Withdrawal Questionnaire, and referral to a substance use disorder (SUD) specialist should be strongly considered, as successful treatment of withdrawal symptoms can predict longer-term treatment outcomes [114]. Symptoms are typically treated with supportive measures, and there are no FDA-approved therapies for this indication.

Chronic Use and Impact on Critical Illness

Chronic effects of stimulants on the heart include myocarditis, dilated cardiomyopathy, and reduced left ventricular systolic function [115]. Systolic function improves significantly with abstinence, but recurrence is associated with relapse [115, 116]. Furthermore, substance use is an independent predictor of emergency department visits and hospitalization in patients with heart failure (HF) [115, 116]. Despite a lower incidence of in-hospital mortality, stimulant-related HF hospitalizations have been associated with increased in-hospital complications such as cardiogenic shock, VT, the need for vasopressors, pulmonary embolism, and AKI [117]. A discussion of the considerations for managing enduring cardiomyopathy and HF in non-abstaining stimulant users, therefore, is warranted.

Standard goal-directed medical therapy (GDMT) should be initiated in patients who continue to use stimulants [115]. As discussed earlier, BBT has traditionally been avoided in cocaine users despite being a mainstay of treatment for ischemic cardiac disease, HF, and cardiomyopathy [118]. A retrospective study comparing the use of BBT in patients using cocaine to abstaining patients revealed no difference in the rates of cardiovascular adverse events and all-cause mortality [119]. A second study found reduced 30-day hospital readmission rates in the group receiving BBT but no difference in all-cause mortality between groups [120]. In another evaluation of patients with cocaine-associated HF and a reduced ejection fraction (EF), a significant reduction in New York Heart Association functional class and improved EF was observed following 12 months of BBT [121, 122]. Collectively, these findings suggest that BBT should be considered in patients with HF who continue to use cocaine, especially if careful consideration is given to selecting a BB with alpha activity. Carvedilol, for example, was associated with a 33% lower rate of major adverse cardiac events in cocaine-use disorder patients with a left ventricular EF $\leq 40\%$ [123]. Current AHA/ACC/Heart Failure Society of America guidelines fail to recommend a specific BB in patients with ongoing cocaine use, and many clinicians may continue to avoid BBT [118]. Some have suggested the routine use of BBT with ongoing cocaine use in all patients except those with recent acute coronary syndromes, uncontrolled hypertension, and/or stroke [78].

Recent evaluations suggest that a treatment approach of GDMT plus stimulant cessation alone is associated with poor outcomes [124]. Increased catecholamine concentrations or repeated episodes of myocarditis may lead to subendocardial ischemia and fibrosis, as well as myocyte necrosis [124]. The irreversible myocyte damage that results can lead to subsequent loss of contractility and dilated cardiomyopathy [115, 120]. Patients with nonischemic cardiomyopathy who continue to use stimulants are more likely to experience substance-induced cardiomyopathy [125]. The decision to pursue advanced mechanical therapy or a heart transplant in the non-abstaining patient, therefore, is complex but warrants consideration. It should be acknowledged that implicit biases regarding substance use disorders may impact clinical decision-making [126]. A major reservation is the concern for infective endocarditis in patients who continue to use injectable substances [125]. Increased rates of leaving against medical advice for stimulant use in patients with heart failure demonstrate cause for concerns about the inability to follow through on plans of care and outpatient follow-up [126]. Patients with substance use disorders may lack insight into their health and have poor medication adherence and/or negative attitudes toward pharmacologic management [125, 126]. Furthermore, in patients experiencing homelessness, lacking social support, or living with concomitant psychiatric illnesses, the concern for their ability and access to care after device implantation or transplant is heightened [125].

Despite a lack of evidence to suggest that implantable cardioverter defibrillators (ICDs) reduce the risk of mortality in stimulant users with or without cardiomyopathy and for primary or secondary prevention in the absence of cardiovascular disease, these devices can be considered for patients with substance-induced cardiomyopathy. The absence of myocardial edema and fibrosis on cardiac magnetic resonance imaging is associated with the potential for functional recovery and can aid in the consideration of whether patients would benefit from ICDs [127]. Further complicating the decision to implant an ICD is the association between phantom shocks, previous electrical storms, and stimulant use [128]. Cocaine has been associated with inappropriate ICD shocks due to the sinus tachycardia brought on by acute use in an apparent time-dependent fashion. In one case, a patient with an ICD presented with VT/VF storm and multiple failed ICD shocks 16 hours after cocaine use [129]. Threshold testing four days later, however, revealed successful defibrillation at half the energy of failed shocks during active cocaine use. Establishing defibrillation thresholds is, therefore, more complex to avoid treatment futility and the increased risk of repeated shocks. In previous studies of substance-associated cardiomyopathies, defibrillation thresholds were approximately 10 joules higher and 13 joules higher in patients with methamphetamine and cocaine use, respectively [130–132]. Lastly, if the decision is made to pursue ICD implantation, establishing adequate follow-up is essential.

Heart transplantation is widely recognized as a life-saving modality to manage end-stage cardiomyopathy [133]. Due to the concern for post-transplantation noncompliance, graft rejection, and low survival rates, most transplant centers require abstinence for a minimum of 6 months prior to considering transplantation in recipients with substance use disorders [133]. Data regarding long-term survival in heart transplant recipients with a history of substance use disorder is limited. Available evidence comparing post-transplantation outcomes in patients with a history of a substance use disorder to those without suggests that despite recipients with a history of a substance use disorder having a higher prevalence of noncompliance and deaths due to noncompliance, there is no difference in overall survival rate [133]. It should be noted, however, that a downward trend in survival rates was observed after posttransplant year three, which may be explained by a relapse in substance use.

Left ventricular assist devices (LVADs) are an option as destination therapy, bridge-to-transplant, or as a bridge-to-recovery strategy, but the evidence to support this is conflicting [134]. While one retrospective evaluation found no significant correlation between preoperative psychosocial risk factors including SUD and readmissions, length of stay, LVAD durability, or mortality, other reviews found an association between active substance use at the time of implantation and greater risk of readmissions from LVAD complications, driveline infections, and mortality [135–137]. Causes of death included LVAD driveline-related sepsis, LVAD thromboses, intracranial hemorrhage attributed to mycotic aneurysms secondary to untreated bacteremia, and multisystem organ failure [137]. This study also found a 69% lower rate of patients in the substance use disorder group being listed for transplant and an 89% lower rate of receiving a transplant, with issues related to noncompliance and ongoing substance use being cited as reasons for not being listed [137]. There is limited evidence to suggest that LVADs can be used as a bridge-to-recovery strategy. Though limited to one case series, the successful use of LVADs in two patients with severe dilated cardiomyopathy associated with amphetamine use as a bridge-to-recovery strategy has been reported. Because both patients were successfully weaned from their LVADs, the authors suggest that amphetamine-associated cardiomyopathy should be considered a reversible cause of HF [124].

While many transplant programs require full abstinence before proceeding with transplant, not all LVAD programs consider active substance use disorder to be an absolute contraindication to device implantation [134]. Guidelines on LVAD patient selection consider ongoing substance abuse to be a relative contraindication and leave the decision of requiring abstinence up to each LVAD program [138]. Some programs, therefore, proceed with LVAD implantation, provided patients are willing to seek post-operative substance use disorder treatment [134]. Treating substance use disorders in patients with LVADs should ideally follow the standard of care and may require inpatient admission to a substance use disorder treatment and rehabilitation center [134]. Admission to these centers may pose a challenge for patients with LVADs, as most centers are ill-equipped or staff have insufficient training to handle the complexity of LVAD maintenance [134]. Because poor maintenance can result in device malfunction or failure, safe admission to a substance use disorder facility would require staff competence in LVAD care. Thus, substance use disorder treatment may need to be carried out in the outpatient setting in patients who are both autonomous enough to manage their LVAD and physically and cognitively capable of participating in outpatient therapy [134].

References

1. Suen LW, Davy-Mendez T, LeSaint KT, Riley ED, Coffin PO. Emergency department visits and trends related to cocaine, psychostimulants, and opioids in the United States, 2008-2018. BMC Emerg Med. 2022;22(1):19. Jones C, Olsen E, O'Donnell J, Mustaquim D. Resurgent methamphetamine use at treatment admission in the United States, 2008–2017. Am J Public Health. 2020;110(4):509–16. https://doi.org/10.2105/ajph.2019.305527.
2. Vivolo-Kantor AM, Hoots BE, Seth P, Jones CM. Recent trends and associated factors of amphetamine-type stimulant overdoses in emergency departments. Drug Alcohol Depend. 2020;216:108323. Hoots B, Vivolo-Kantor A, Seth P. The rise in non-fatal and fatal overdoses involving stimulants with and without opioids in the United States. Addiction. 2020;115(5):946–958. https://doi.org/10.1111/add.14878.
3. Substance Abuse and Mental Health Services Administration. Key substance use and mental health indicators in the United States: results from the 2021 National Survey on Drug Use and Health (HHS Publication No. PEP22-07-01-005, NSDUH Series H-57). Center for Behavioral Health Statistics and Quality, Substance Abuse and Mental Health Services Administration. 2022. Available from: https://www.samhsa.gov/data/report/2021-nsduh-annual-national-report
4. United Nations Office on Drugs and Crime. World drug report 2022: drug market trends cocaine amphetamine-type stimulants new psychoactive substances. In: United Nations publication. 2022. Available from: https://www.unodc/org/unodc/en/data-and-analysis/world-drug-report-2022.html
5. Hoopsick RA, Yockey RA. Methamphetamine-related mortality in the United States: co-involvement of Heroin and Fentanyl, 1999–2021. Am J Pub Health. 2023;113(4):416–9.
6. Haddad LM. 1978: cocaine in perspective. JACEP. 1979;8(9):374–6. https://doi.org/10.1016/s0361-1124(79)80263-4.
7. Knuepfer MM. Cardiovascular disorders associated with cocaine use: myths and truths. Pharmacol Ther. 2003;97(3):181–222. https://doi.org/10.1016/s0163-7258(02)00329-7.
8. Johanson CE, Fischman MW. The pharmacology of cocaine related to its abuse. Pharmacol Rev. 1989;41(1):3–52.
9. Siegel RK. Cocaine smoking. N Engl J Med. 1979;300(7):373. https://doi.org/10.1056/NEJM197902153000731.
10. Coleman DL, Ross TF, Naughton JL. Myocardial ischemia and infarction related to recreational cocaine use. West J Med. 1982;136(5):444–6.
11. United Nations Office on Drugs and Crime. Global report on cocaine 2023 – local dynamics, global challenges. United Nations; 2023. Available from: https://www.unodc.org/documents/data-and-analysis/cocaine/Global_cocaine_report_2023.pdf
12. Heal DJ, Smith SL, Gosden J, Nutt DJ. Amphetamine, past and present–a pharmacological and clinical perspective. J Psychopharmacol. 2013;27(6):479–96. https://doi.org/10.1177/0269881113482532.
13. Bett WR. Benzedrine sulphate in clinical medicine; a survey of the literature. Postgrad Med J. 1946;22(250):205–18. https://doi.org/10.1136/pgmj.22.250.205.
14. Khoramizadeh M, Effatpanah M, Mostaghimi A, Rezaei M, Mahjoub A, Shishehgar S. Treatment of amphetamine abuse/use disorder: a systematic review of a recent health concern. Daru. 2019;27(2):743–53. https://doi.org/10.1007/s40199-019-00282-3.
15. Kuropka P, Zawadzki M, Szpot. A narrative review of the neuropharmacology of synthetic cathinones – popular alternatives to classical drugs of abuse. Hum Psychopharmacol Clin Exp. 2023;38:e2866. https://doi.org/10.1002/hup.2866.
16. Drug Enforcement Administration. Drugs of abuse, a DEA resource guide: 2020 edition. 2020. Available from: https://www.dea.gov/sites/default/files/2020-04/Drugs%20of%20Abuse%202020-Web%20Version-508%20compliant-4-24-20_0.pdf
17. Kalix P. Cathinone, a natural amphetamine. Pharmacol Toxicol. 1992;70(2):77–86. https://doi.org/10.1111/j.1600-0773.1992.tb00434.x.

18. Shafi A, Berry AJ, Sumnall H, Wood DM, Tracy DK. New psychoactive substance: a review and updates. Ther Adv Psychopharmacol. 2020;10:2045125320967197. https://doi.org/10.1177/2045125320967197.
19. Bijlsma L, Bade R, Been F, Celma A, Castiglioni S. Perspectives and challenges associated with determination of new psychoactive substances in urine and wastewater – a tutorial. Anal Chim Acta. 2021;1145:132–47. https://doi.org/10.1016/j.aca.2020.08.058.
20. Hyde JF, Browning E, Adams R. Synthetic homologs of d,l-ephedrine. J Am Chem Soc. 1928;50(8):2287–92. https://doi.org/10.1021/ja01395a032.
21. Krotulski AJ, Walton SE, Mohr ALA, Logan BK. NPS discovery Q1 2023 trend reports. United States: Center for Forensic Science Research and Education; 2023. Available from: https://www.cfsre.org/images/trendreports/2023_Q1_CFSRE_NPS_Discovery_Trend_Reports.pdf
22. German CL, Fleckenstein AE, Hanson GR. Bath salts and synthetic cathinones: an emerging designer drug phenomenon. Life Sci. 2014;97(1):2–8. https://doi.org/10.1016/j.lfs.2013.07.023.
23. Egashira K, Morgan KG, Morgan JP. Effects of cocaine on excitation-contraction coupling of aortic smooth muscle from the ferret. J Clin Invest. 1991;87(4):1322–8. https://doi.org/10.1172/JCI115135.
24. Jones SR, Garris PA, Wightman RM. Different effects of cocaine and nomifensine on dopamine uptake in the caudate-putamen and nucleus accumbens. J Pharmacol Exp Ther. 1995;274(1):396–403.
25. Venton BJ, Seipel AT, Phillips PE, Wetsel WC, Gitler D, Greengard P, Augustine GJ, Wightman RM. Cocaine increases dopamine release by mobilization of a synapsin-dependent reserve pool. J Neurosci. 2006;26(12):3206–9. https://doi.org/10.1523/JNEUROSCI.4901-04.2006.
26. Lange RA, Cigarroa RG, Yancy CW Jr, Willard JE, Popma JJ, Sills MN, McBride W, Kim AS, Hillis LD. Cocaine-induced coronary-artery vasoconstriction. N Engl J Med. 1989;321(23):1557–62. https://doi.org/10.1056/NEJM198912073212301.
27. Moliterno DJ, Lange RA, Gerard RD, Willard JE, Lackner C, Hillis LD. Influence of intranasal cocaine on plasma constituents associated with endogenous thrombosis and thrombolysis. Am J Med. 1994;96(6):492–6. https://doi.org/10.1016/0002-9343(94)90087-6.
28. Liaudet L, Calderari B, Pacher P. Pathophysiological mechanisms of catecholamine and cocaine-mediated cardiotoxicity. Heart Fail Rev. 2014;19(6):815–24. https://doi.org/10.1007/s10741-014-9418-y.
29. O'Leary ME, Hancox JC. Role of voltage-gated sodium, potassium and calcium channels in the development of cocaine-associated cardiac arrhythmias. Br J Clin Pharmacol. 2010;69(5):427–42. https://doi.org/10.1111/j.1365-2125.2010.03629.x.
30. Om A, Ellenbogen KA, Vetrovec GW. Cocaine-induced bradyarrhythmias. Am Heart J. 1992;124(1):232–4. https://doi.org/10.1016/0002-8703(92)90952-r.
31. Franklin SM, Thihalolipavan S, Fontaine JM. Sinus bradycardia in habitual cocaine users. Am J Cardiol. 2017;119(10):1611–5. https://doi.org/10.1016/j.amjcard.2017.02.018.
32. Chen LC, Graefe JF, Shojaie J, Willetts J, Wood RW. Pulmonary effects of the cocaine pyrolysis product, methylecgonidine, in guinea pigs. Life Sci. 1995;56(1):PL7–12. https://doi.org/10.1016/0024-3205(94)00410-t.
33. Ettinger NA, Albin RJ. A review of the respiratory effects of smoking cocaine. Am J Med. 1989;87(6):664–8. https://doi.org/10.1016/s0002-9343(89)80401-2.
34. Smollin C, Hoffman R. Cocaine. In: Nelson L, Howland M, Lewin N, Smith S, Goldfrank L, Hoffman R, et al., editors. Goldfrank's toxicologic emergencies, 11e. New York: McGraw-Hill Education; 2019.
35. Jeffcoat AR, Perez-Reyes M, Hill JM, Sadler BM, Cook CE. Cocaine disposition in humans after intravenous injection, nasal insufflation (snorting), or smoking. Drug Metab Dispos. 1989;17(2):153–9.
36. Van Dyke C, Jatlow P, Ungerer J, Barash PG, Byck R. Oral cocaine: plasma concentrations and central effects. Science. 1978;200(4338):211–3. https://doi.org/10.1126/science.24895.

37. Stewart DJ, Inaba T, Lucassen M, Kalow W. Cocaine metabolism: cocaine and norcocaine hydrolysis by liver and serum esterases. Clin Pharmacol Ther. 1979;25(4):464–8. https://doi.org/10.1002/cpt1979254464.
38. O'Leary ME. Inhibition of HERG potassium channels by cocaethylene: a metabolite of cocaine and ethanol. Cardiovasc Res. 2002;53(1):59–67. https://doi.org/10.1016/s0008-6363(01)00458-8.
39. Scheidweiler KB, Plessinger MA, Shojaie J, Wood RW, Kwong TC. Pharmacokinetics and pharmacodynamics of methylecgonidine, a crack cocaine pyrolyzate. J Pharmacol Exp Ther. 2003;307(3):1179–87. https://doi.org/10.1124/jpet.103.055434.
40. Marzuk PM, Tardiff K, Leon AC, Hirsch CS, Portera L, Iqbal MI, Nock MK, Hartwell N. Ambient temperature and mortality from unintentional cocaine overdose. JAMA. 1998;279(22):1795–800. https://doi.org/10.1001/jama.279.22.1795.
41. Olson KR, Pentel PR, Kelley MT. Physical assessment and differential diagnosis of the poisoned patient. Med Toxicol. 1987;2(1):52–81. https://doi.org/10.1007/BF03259860.
42. Levine SL, Brust JCM, Futrell N, Ho KL, Blake D, Millikan CH, Brass LM, Fayad P, Schultz LR, Selwa JF, Welch KMA. Cerebrovascular complications of the use of the "crack" form of alkaloidal cocaine. N Engl J Med. 1990;323(11):699–704. https://doi.org/10.1056/NEJM199009133231102.
43. Mangiardi JR, Daras M, Geller ME, Weitzner I, Tuchman AJ. Cocaine-related intracranial hemorrhage. Report of nine cases and review. Acta Neurol Scand. 1988;77(3):177–80. https://doi.org/10.1111/j.1600-0404.1988.tb05891.x.
44. Daras M, Tuchman AJ, Marks S. Central nervous system infarction related to cocaine abuse. Stroke. 1991;22(10):1320–5. https://doi.org/10.1161/01.str.22.10.1320.
45. Riezzo I, Fiore C, De Carlo D, Pascale N, Neri M, Turillazzi E, Fineschi V. Side effects of cocaine abuse: multiorgan toxicity and pathological consequences. Curr Med Chem. 2012;19(33):5624–46. https://doi.org/10.2174/092986712803988893.
46. Ruttenber AJ, McAnally HB, Wetli CV. Cocaine-associated rhabdomyolysis and excited delirium: different stages of the same syndrome. Am J Forensic Med Pathol. 1999;20(2):120–7. https://doi.org/10.1097/00000433-199906000-00003.
47. Brady KT, Lydiard RB, Malcolm R, Ballenger JC. Cocaine-induced psychosis. J Clin Psychiatry. 1991;52(12):509–12.
48. Daras M, Koppel BS, Atos-Radzion E. Cocaine-induced choreoathetoid movements ('crack dancing'). Neurology. 1994;44(4):751–2. https://doi.org/10.1212/wnl.44.4.751.
49. Hoffman RS, Reimer BS. "Crack" cocaine-induced bilateral amblyopia. Am J Emerg Med. 1993;11(1):35–7. https://doi.org/10.1016/0735-6757(93)90055-g.
50. Libman RB, Masters SR, de Paola A, Mohr JP. Transient monocular blindness associated with cocaine abuse. Neurology. 1993;43(1):228–9. https://doi.org/10.1212/wnl.43.1_part_1.228-a.
51. Niazi M, Kondru A, Levy J, Bloom AA. Spectrum of ischemic colitis in cocaine users. Dig Dis Sci. 1997;42(7):1537–41. https://doi.org/10.1023/a:1018839415743.
52. Freudenberger RS, Cappell MS, Hutt DA. Intestinal infarction after intravenous cocaine administration. Ann Intern Med. 1990;113(9):715–6. https://doi.org/10.7326/0003-4819-113-9-715.
53. Edmondson DA, Towne JB, Foley DW, Abu-Hajir M, Kochar MS. Cocaine-induced renal artery dissection and thrombosis leading to renal infarction. WMJ. 2004;103(7):66–9.
54. Gold M, Boyack I, Caputo N, Pearlman A. Imaging prevalence of nasal septal perforation in an urban population. Clin Imaging. 2017;43:80–2. https://doi.org/10.1016/j.clinimag.2017.02.002.
55. Kudrow DB, Henry DA, Haake DA, Marshall G, Mathisen GE. Botulism associated with Clostridium botulinum sinusitis after intranasal cocaine abuse. Ann Intern Med. 1988;109(12):984–5. https://doi.org/10.7326/0003-4819-109-12-984.
56. Counselman FL, McLaughlin EW, Kardon EM, Bhambhani-Bhavnani AS. Creatine phosphokinase elevation in patients presenting to the emergency department with cocaine-related complaints. Am J Emerg Med. 1997;15(3):221–3. https://doi.org/10.1016/s0735-6757(97)90000-0.

57. Marzuk PM, Tardiff K, Leon AC, Hirsch CS, Stajic M, Portera L, Hartwell N, Iqbal MI. Fatal injuries after cocaine use as a leading cause of death among young adults in New York City. N Engl J Med. 1995;332(26):1753–7. https://doi.org/10.1056/NEJM199506293322606.
58. Collins CG, Seoighe D, Ireland A, Bouchier-Hayes D, McGrath F. Cocaine-associated lower limb ischemia. Vascular. 2008;16(5):297–9. https://doi.org/10.2310/6670.2008.00048.
59. McMullin CM, Bayat I, Rytina E, See TC, Varty K, Coughlin PA. Profound acute limb ischemia affecting all four limbs following cocaine inhalation. J Vasc Surg. 2015;61(2):504–6. https://doi.org/10.1016/j.jvs.2013.09.010.
60. Brady WJ Jr, Duncan CW. Hypoglycemia masquerading as acute psychosis and acute cocaine intoxication. Am J Emerg Med. 1999;17(3):318–9. https://doi.org/10.1016/s0735-6757(99)90140-7.
61. Schwartz BG, Rezkalla S, Kloner RA. Cardiovascular effects of cocaine. Circulation. 2010;122(24):2558–69. https://doi.org/10.1161/CIRCULATIONAHA.110.940569.
62. Lange RA, Hillis LD. Cardiovascular complications of cocaine use. N Engl J Med. 2001;345(5):351–8. https://doi.org/10.1056/NEJM200108023450507.
63. Bauman JL, Grawe JJ, Winecoff AP, Hariman RJ. Cocaine-related sudden cardiac death: a hypothesis correlating basic science and clinical observations. J Clin Pharmacol. 1994;34(9):902–11. https://doi.org/10.1002/j.1552-4604.1994.tb04003.x.
64. Mittleman MA, Mintzer D, Maclure M, Tofler GH, Sherwood JB, Muller JE. Triggering of myocardial infarction by cocaine. Circulation. 1999;99(21):2737–41. https://doi.org/10.1161/01.cir.99.21.2737.
65. Tames SM, Goldenring JM. Madarosis from cocaine use. N Engl J Med. 1986;314(20):1324. https://doi.org/10.1056/nejm198605153142020.
66. Castro-Villamor MA, de las Heras P, Armentia A, Dueñas-Laita A. Cocaine-induced severe angioedema and urticaria. Ann Emerg Med. 1999;34(2):296–7. https://doi.org/10.1016/s0196-0644(99)70257-x.
67. Cohen ME, Kegel JG. Candy cocaine esophagus. Chest. 2002;121(5):1701–3. https://doi.org/10.1378/chest.121.5.1701.
68. Restrepo CS, Carrillo JA, Martínez S, Ojeda P, Rivera AL, Hatta A. Pulmonary complications from cocaine and cocaine-based substances: imaging manifestations. Radiographics. 2007;27(4):941–56. https://doi.org/10.1148/rg.274065144.
69. Jatlow P, Barash PG, Van Dyke C, Radding J, Byck R. Cocaine and succinylcholine sensitivity: a new caution. Anesth Analg. 1979;58(3):235–8.
70. Plane AF, Marsan PE, du Cheyron D, Valette X. Rapidly changing ECG in hyperkalaemia after succinylcholine. Lancet. 2019;393(10184):1983. https://doi.org/10.1016/S0140-6736(19)30838-4.
71. Laskowski LK, Landry A, Vassallo SU, Hoffman RS. Ice water submersion for rapid cooling in severe drug-induced hyperthermia. Clin Toxicol (Phila). 2015;53(3):181–4. https://doi.org/10.3109/15563650.2015.1009994.
72. Fox AW. More on rhabdomyolysis associated with cocaine intoxication. N Engl J Med. 1989;321(18):1271. https://doi.org/10.1056/nejm198911023211818.
73. Heard K, Cleveland NR, Krier S. Benzodiazepines and antipsychotic medications for treatment of acute cocaine toxicity in animal models--a systematic review and meta-analysis. Hum Exp Toxicol. 2011;30(11):1849–54. https://doi.org/10.1177/0960327111401435.
74. Elkattawy S, Alyacoub R, Al-Nassarei A, Younes I, Ayad S, Habib M. Cocaine induced heart failure: report and literature review. J Community Hosp Intern Med Perspect. 2021;11(4):547–50. https://doi.org/10.1080/20009666.2021.1926614.
75. Kontak AC, Victor RG, Vongpatanasin W. Dexmedetomidine as a novel countermeasure for cocaine-induced central sympathoexcitation in cocaine-addicted humans. Hypertension. 2013;61(2):388–94. https://doi.org/10.1161/HYPERTENSIONAHA.112.203554.
76. Chan GM, Sharma R, Price D, Hoffman RS, Nelson LS. Phentolamine therapy for cocaine-association acute coronary syndrome (CAACS). J Med Toxicol. 2006;2(3):108–11. https://doi.org/10.1007/BF03161019.

77. Richards JR, Garber D, Laurin EG, Albertson TE, Derlet RW, Amsterdam EA, Olson KR, Ramoska EA, Lange RA. Treatment of cocaine cardiovascular toxicity: a systematic review. Clin Toxicol (Phila). 2016;54(5):345–64. https://doi.org/10.3109/15563650.2016.
78. Littmann L, Narveson SY, Fesel NM, Marconi SL. Beta blocker treatment of heart failure patients with ongoing cocaine use. Int J Cardiol. 2013;168(3):2919–20. https://doi.org/10.1016/j.ijcard.2013.03.187.
79. Lo KB, Virk HUH, Lakhter V, Ram P, Gongora C, Pressman G, Figueredo V. Clinical outcomes after treatment of cocaine-induced chest pain with beta-blockers: a systematic review and meta-analysis. Am J Med. 2019;132(4):505–9. https://doi.org/10.1016/j.amjmed.2018.11.041.
80. Amsterdam EA, Wenger NK, Brindis RG, Casey DE Jr, Ganiats TG, Holmes DR Jr, Jaffe AS, Jneid H, Kelly RF, Kontos MC, Levine GN, Liebson PR, Mukherjee D, Peterson ED, Sabatine MS, Smalling RW, Zieman SJ, ACC/AHA Task Force Members. 2014 AHA/ACC guideline for the management of patients with non-ST-elevation acute coronary syndromes: a report of the American College of Cardiology/American Heart Association Task Force on Practice Guidelines. Circulation. 2014;130(25):e344–426. https://doi.org/10.1161/CIR.0000000000000134.
81. Kalimullah EA, Bryant SM. Case files of the medical toxicology fellowship at the toxikon consortium in Chicago: cocaine-associated wide-complex dysrhythmias and cardiac arrest – treatment nuances and controversies. J Med Toxicol. 2008;4(4):277–83. https://doi.org/10.1007/BF03161213.
82. 2005 American Heart Association Guidelines for cardiopulmonary resuscitation and emergency cardiovascular care. Part 10.2: toxicology in ECC. Circulation 2005;112:Suppl IV-126–IV-132.
83. McCord J, Jneid H, Hollander JE, de Lemos JA, Cercek B, Hsue P, Gibler WB, Ohman EM, Drew B, Philippides G, Newby LK. American Heart Association Acute Cardiac Care Committee of the Council on Clinical Cardiology. Management of cocaine-associated chest pain and myocardial infarction: a scientific statement from the American Heart Association Acute Cardiac Care Committee of the Council on Clinical Cardiology. Circulation. 2008;117(14):1897–907. https://doi.org/10.1161/CIRCULATIONAHA.107.188950.
84. Spyres M, Jang D. Amphetamines. In: Nelson L, Howland M, Lewin N, Smith S, Goldfrank L, Hoffman R, editors. Goldfrank's Toxicologic Emergencies, 11e. McGraw Hill; 2019.
85. Baig AM. DARK side of amphetamine and analogues: Pharmacology, syndromic manifestation, and management of amphetamine addiction. ACS Chem Neurosci. 2018;9(10):2299–303. https://doi.org/10.1021/acschemneuro.8b00137.
86. Cruickshank CC, Dyer KR. A review of the clinical pharmacology of methamphetamine. Addiction. 2009;104(7):1085–99. https://doi.org/10.1111/j.1360-0443.2009.02564.x.
87. Allain F, Minogianis EA, Roberts DC, Samaha AN. How fast and how often: the pharmacokinetics of drug use are decisive in addiction. Neurosci Biobehav Rev. 2015;56:166–79. https://doi.org/10.1016/j.neubiorev.2015.06.012.
88. Hart CL, Gunderson EW, Perez A, Kirkpatrick MG, Thurmond A, Comer SD, Foltin RW. Acute physiological and behavioral effects of intranasal methamphetamine in humans. Neuropsychopharmacology. 2008;33(8):1847–55. https://doi.org/10.1038/sj.npp.1301578.
89. Derlet RW, Rice P, Horowitz BZ, Lord RV. Amphetamine toxicity: experience with 127 cases. J Emerg Med. 1989;7:157–61. https://doi.org/10.1016/0736-4679(89)90263-1.
90. Kaye S, McKetin R, Duflou J, Darke S. Methamphetamine and cardiovascular pathology: a review of the evidence. Addiction. 2007;102(8):1204–11. https://doi.org/10.1111/j.1360-0443.2007.01874.x.
91. Hung YM, Chang JC. Weight-reducing regimen associated with polymorphic ventricular tachycardia. Am J Emerg Med. 2006;24(6):714–6. https://doi.org/10.1016/j.ajem.2006.02.004.
92. McGee SM, McGee DN, McGee MB. Spontaneous intracerebral hemorrhage related to methamphetamine abuse: autopsy findings and clinical correlation. Am J Forensic Med Pathol. 2004;25(4):334–7. https://doi.org/10.1097/01.paf.0000137206.16785.2f.

93. Möller M, Völz J, Paliege R, Lenz C, Gradaus R, Neuzner J. Ecstasy-induced myocardial infarction in a teenager: rare complication of a widely used illicit drug. Clin Res Cardiol. 2010;99(12):849–51. https://doi.org/10.1007/s00392-010-0205-z.
94. Westover AN, Nakonezny PA. Aortic dissection in young adults who abuse amphetamines. Am Heart J. 2010;160(2):315–21. https://doi.org/10.1016/j.ahj.2010.05.021.
95. Holubar SD, Hassinger JP, Dozois EJ, Masuoka HC. Methamphetamine colitis: a rare case of ischemic colitis in a young patient. Arch Surg. 2009;144(8):780–2. https://doi.org/10.1001/archsurg.2009.139.
96. Isoardi KZ, Mudge DW, Harris K, Dimeski G, Buckley NA. Methamphetamine intoxication and acute kidney injury: a prospective observational case series. Nephrology (Carlton). 2020;25(10):758–64. https://doi.org/10.1111/nep.13762.
97. Eilert RJ, Kliewer ML. Methamphetamine-induced rhabdomyolysis. Int Anesthesiol Clin. 2011;49(2):52–6. https://doi.org/10.1097/AIA.0b013e3181ffc0e5.
98. Kendrick WC, Hull AR, Knochel JP. Rhabdomyolysis and shock after intravenous amphetamine administration. Ann Intern Med. 1977;86(4):381–7. https://doi.org/10.7326/0003-4819-86-4-381.
99. Richards JR, Placone TW, Wang CG, van der Linden MC, Derlet RW, Laurin EG. Methamphetamine, amphetamine, and MDMA use and emergency department recidivism. J Emerg Med. 2020;59(2):320–8. https://doi.org/10.1016/j.jemermed.2020.04.051.
100. Zhu BL, Oritani S, Shimotouge K, Ishida K, Quan L, Fujita MQ, Ogawa M, Maeda H. Methamphetamine-related fatalities in forensic autopsy during 5 years in the southern half of Osaka city and surrounding areas. Forensic Sci Int. 2000;113(1–3):443–7. https://doi.org/10.1016/s0379-0738(00)00281-4.
101. Richards JR, Derlet RW, Duncan DR. Chemical restraint for the agitated patient in the emergency department: lorazepam versus droperidol. J Emerg Med. 1998;16(4):567–73. https://doi.org/10.1016/s0736-4679(98)00045-6.
102. Barbic D, Andolfatto G, Grunau B, Scheuermeyer FX, Macewan B, Qian H, Wong H, Barbic SP, Honer W. Rapid agitation control with ketamine in the emergency department: a blinded, randomized controlled trial. Ann Emerg Med. 2021;78(6):788–95. https://doi.org/10.1016/j.annemergmed.2021.05.023.
103. Grunau BE, Wiens MO, Brubacher JR. Dantrolene in the treatment of MDMA-related hyperpyrexia: a systematic review. CJEM. 2010;12(5):435–42. https://doi.org/10.1017/s1481803500012598.
104. Curry SC, Chang D, Connor D. Drug- and toxin-induced rhabdomyolysis. Ann Emerg Med. 1989;18(10):1068–84. https://doi.org/10.1016/s0196-0644(89)80933-3.
105. Hegadoren KM, Baker GB, Bourin M. 3,4-Methylenedioxy analogues of amphetamine: defining the risks to humans. Neurosci Biobehav Rev. 1999;23(4):539–53. https://doi.org/10.1016/s0149-7634(98)00046-3.
106. de la Torre R, Farré M, Roset P, Pizarro N, Abanades S, Segura M, Segura J, Camí J. Human pharmacology of MDMA: pharmacokinetics, metabolism, and disposition. Ther Drug Monit. 2004;26(2):137–44. https://doi.org/10.1097/00007691-200404000-00009.
107. Ghatol A, Kazory A. Ecstasy-associated acute severe hyponatremia and cerebral edema: a role for osmotic diuresis? J Emerg Med. 2012;42(6):e137–40. https://doi.org/10.1016/j.jemermed.2009.05.001.
108. Sporer KA, Lesser SH. Cocaine washed-out syndrome. Ann Emerg Med. 1992;21(1):112. https://doi.org/10.1016/s0196-0644(05)82275-9.
109. Trabulsy ME. Cocaine washed out syndrome in a patient with acute myocardial infarction. Am J Emerg Med. 1995;13(5):538–9. https://doi.org/10.1016/0735-6757(95)90166-3.
110. Bolds M. Substance use disorder in critical care. Crit Care Nurs Clin Am. 2023; Epub ahead of print. https://doi.org/10.1016/j.cnc.2023.06.004
111. McGregor C, Srisurapanont M, Jittiwutikarn J, Laobhripatr S, Wongtan T, White JM. The nature, time course and severity of methamphetamine withdrawal. Addiction. 2005;100(9):1320–9. https://doi.org/10.1111/j.1360-0443.2005.01160.x.
112. Watson R, Hartmann E, Schildkraut JJ. Amphetamine withdrawal: affective state, sleep patterns, and MHPG excretion. Am J Psychiatry. 1972;129(3):263–9. https://doi.org/10.1176/ajp.129.3.263.

113. Shoptaw SJ, Kao U, Heinzerling K, Ling W. Treatment for amphetamine withdrawal. Cochrane Database Syst Rev. 2009;2009(2):CD003021. https://doi.org/10.1002/14651858.CD003021.pub2.
114. Brecht ML, von Mayrhauser C, Anglin MD. Predictors of relapse after treatment for methamphetamine use. J Psychoactive Drugs. 2000;32(2):211–20. https://doi.org/10.1080/02791072.2000.10400231.
115. Grubb AF, Greene SJ, Fudim M, Dewald T, Mentz RJ. Drugs of abuse and heart failure. J Card Fail. 2021;27(11):1260–75. https://doi.org/10.1016/j.cardfail.2021.05.023.
116. Hollander JE, Hoffman RS, Gennis P, Fairweather P, Feldman JA, Fish SS, DiSano MJ, Schumb DA, Dyer S. Cocaine-associated chest pain: one-year follow-up. Acad Emerg Med. 1995;2(3):179–84. https://doi.org/10.1111/j.1553-2712.1995.tb03191.x.
117. Shetty S, Malik AH, Ali A, Yang YC, Briasoulis A, Alvarez P. Characteristics, trends, outcomes, and costs of stimulant-related acute heart failure hospitalizations in the United States. Int J Cardiol. 2021;331:158–63. https://doi.org/10.1016/j.ijcard.2021.01.060.
118. Heidenreich PA, Bozkurt B, Aguilar D, Allen LA, Byun JJ, Colvin MM, Deswal A, Drazner MH, Dunlay SM, Evers LR, Fang JC, Fedson SE, Fonarow GC, Hayek SS, Hernandez AF, Khazanie P, Kittleson MM, Lee CS, Link MS, Milano CA, Nnacheta LC, Sandhu AT, Stevenson LW, Vardeny O, Vest AR, Yancy CW. 2022 AHA/ACC/HFSA guideline for the management of heart failure: a report of the American College of Cardiology/American Heart Association joint committee on clinical practice guidelines. Circulation. 2022;145(18):e895–e1032. https://doi.org/10.1161/CIR.0000000000001063.
119. Nguyen P, Kamran H, Nasir S, Chan W, Shah T, Deswal A, Bozkurt B. Comparison of frequency of cardiovascular events and mortality in patients with heart failure using versus not using cocaine. Am J Cardiol. 2017;119(12):2030–4. https://doi.org/10.1016/j.amjcard.2017.03.034.
120. Egbuche O, Ekechukwu I, Effoe V, Maduabum N, Millard HR, Maihemuti A, Cross JA, Adedinsewo D, Onwuanyi AE. Effect of β-blocker therapy on hospital readmission and mortality in heart failure patients with concurrent cocaine use. J Cardiovasc Pharmacol Ther. 2018;23(6):518–23. https://doi.org/10.1177/1074248418778550.
121. Lopez PD, Akinlonu A, Mene-Afejuku TO, Dumancas C, Saeed M, Cativo EH, Visco F, Mushiyev S, Pekler G. Clinical outcomes of B-blocker therapy in cocaine-associated heart failure. Int J Cardiol. 2019;277:153–8. https://doi.org/10.1016/j.ijcard.2018.08.058.
122. Lopez P, Akinlonu A, Mene-Afejuku TO, Dumancas C, Saeed M, Cativo EH, Visco F, Mushiyev S, Pekler G. Improvement in clinical outcomes of patients with heart failure and active cocaine use after β-blocker therapy. Clin Cardiol. 2018;41(4):465–9. https://doi.org/10.1002/clc.22897.
123. Banerji D, Alvi RM, Afshar M, Tariq N, Rokicki A, Mulligan CP, Zhang L, Hassan MO, Awadalla M, Groarke JD, Neilan TG. Carvedilol among patients with heart failure with a cocaine-use disorder. JACC Heart Fail. 2019;7(9):771–8. https://doi.org/10.1016/j.jchf.2019.06.010.
124. Soucy-Giguère MC, Cinq-Mars A, Charbonneau É, Voisine P, Beaudoin J, Dubois M, Sénéchal M. Usefulness of left ventricular assist device in the recovery of severe amphetamine-associated dilated cardiomyopathy. Can J Cardiol. 2020;36(2):317.e5–7. https://doi.org/10.1016/j.cjca.2019.09.024.
125. Dominic P, Ahmad J, Awwab H, Bhuiyan MS, Kevil CG, Goeders NE, Murnane K, Patterson J, Sandau KE, Gopinathannair R, Olshansky B. Stimulant drugs of abuse and cardiac arrhythmias. Circ Arrhythm Electrophysiol. 2022;15(1):e010273. https://doi.org/10.1161/CIRCEP.121.010273.
126. Thyagaturu HS, Bolton AR, Li S, Gonuguntla K, Kumar A, Bianco C, Balla S. Effect of cocaine, amphetamine, and cannabis use disorders on 30-day readmissions of patients with heart failure. Curr Probl Cardiol. 2023;48(8):101189. https://doi.org/10.1016/j.cpcardiol.2022.101189.
127. Pujol-López M, Ortega-Paz L, Flores-Umanzor EJ, Perea RJ, Bosch X. Cardiac magnetic resonance as an alternative to endomyocardial biopsy to predict recoverability of left ventricular function in methamphetamine-associated cardiomyopathy. JACC Heart Fail. 2017;5(11):853–4. https://doi.org/10.1016/j.jchf.2017.08.009.

128. Jacob S, Panaich SS, Zalawadiya SK, McKelvey G, Abraham G, Aravindhakshan R, Sears SF, Conti JB, Marsh HM. Phantom shocks unmasked: clinical data and proposed mechanism of memory reactivation of past traumatic shocks in patients with implantable cardioverter defibrillators. J Interv Card Electrophysiol. 2012;34(2):205–13. https://doi.org/10.1007/s10840-011-9640-7.
129. Nishimura M, Bhatia H, Ma J, Dickson SD, Alshawabkeh L, Adler E, Maisel A, Criqui MH, Greenberg B, Thomas IC. The impact of substance abuse on heart failure hospitalizations. Am J Med. 2020;133(2):207–213.e1. https://doi.org/10.1016/j.amjmed.2019.07.017.
130. Malhotra R, Patel S, Ramchand T, Al Nimri O. Higher defibrillation threshold in methamphetamine cardiomyopathy patients with implantable cardioverter-defibrillator. Indian Pacing Electrophysiol J. 2017;17(6):167–70. https://doi.org/10.1016/j.ipej.2017.07.002.
131. Perrine SA, Nayak R, Bharadwaj AS, McKelvey G, Mohamad T, Jacob S. Effect of substance abuse on defibrillation threshold in patients with implantable cardioverter-defibrillator. Pacing Clin Electrophysiol. 2011;34(2):193–9. https://doi.org/10.1111/j.1540-8159.2010.02907.x.
132. Chen J, Naseem RH, Obel O, Joglar JA. Habitual cocaine use is associated with high defibrillation threshold during ICD implantation. J Cardiovasc Electrophysiol. 2007;18(7):722–5. https://doi.org/10.1111/j.1540-8167.2007.00834.x.
133. Hanrahan JS, Eberly C, Mohanty PK. Substance abuse in heart transplant recipients: a 10-year follow-up study. Prog Transplant. 2001;11(4):285–90. https://doi.org/10.1177/152692480101100410.
134. Choi J, Alexis J, Gosev I, Zimbrean P, Nickels M. Management of substance use disorders in a patient with left ventricular assist device. J Acad Consult Liaison Psychiatry. 2021;62(6):568–76. https://doi.org/10.1016/j.jaclp.2021.07.015.
135. Woodhouse K, Lietz K, Branch A, Spruill J, Lewis-McGowan L, McGrath M, Herre J. Relationship between candidate psychosocial risk profile, post-implant medical compliance and clinical outcomes of LVAD therapy [abstract]. J Heart Lung Transplant. 2014;33(4S):S126.
136. Snipelisky D, Stulak JM, Schettle SD, Sharma S, Kushwaha SS, Dunlay SM. Psychosocial characteristics and outcomes in patients with left ventricular assist device implanted as destination therapy. Am Heart J. 2015;170(5):887–94. https://doi.org/10.1016/j.ahj.2015.08.012.
137. Cogswell R, Smith E, Hamel A, Bauman L, Herr A, Duval S, John R, Roman D, Adatya S, Colvin-Adams M, Garry D, Martin C, Missov E, Pritzker M, Roberts J, Eckman P. Substance abuse at the time of left ventricular assist device implantation is associated with increased mortality. J Heart Lung Transplant. 2014;33(10):1048–55. https://doi.org/10.1016/j.healun.2014.06.009.
138. Saeed D, Feldman D, Banayosy AE, Birks E, Blume E, Cowger J, Hayward C, Jorde U, Kremer J, MacGowan G, Maltais S, Maybaum S, Mehra M, Shah KB, Mohacsi P, Schweiger M, Schroeder SE, Shah P, Slepian M, Tops LF, Alvarez P, Arabia F, Aslam S, Benson-Louis L 4th, Birati E, Buchholz HW, Cedars A, Christensen D, Ciarka A, Coglianese E, Cogswell R, Cook J, Copeland J, Costello JG, Drakos SG, Eghtesady P, Elliot T, Estep JD, Eulert-Grehn JJ, Fabrizio R, Garbade J, Gelow J, Guglin M, Hernandez-Montfort J, Horstmanshof D, John R, Kanwar M, Khaliel F, Kim G, Kumar S, Lavee J, Leache M, Leprince P, Lim S, Loforte A, Maly J, Najjar S, Netuka I, Pamboukian SV, Patel SR, Pinney S, Pluym CV, Potapov E, Robson D, Rochlani Y, Russell S, Sandau K, Sandoval E, Sayer G, Schettle S, Schibilsky D, Schlöglhofer T, Schmitto J, Siddique A, Silvestry S, Slaughter MS, Sun B, Takayama H, Tedford R, Teuteberg JJ, Ton VK, Uriel N, Vierecke J, Zimpfer D, D'Alessandro D. The 2023 International Society for Heart and Lung Transplantation guidelines for mechanical circulatory support: A 10-year update. J Heart Lung Transplant. 2023;42(7):e1–e222. https://doi.org/10.1016/j.healun.2022.12.004.

Chapter 9
Psychoactive Medications in the ICU

Sean P. Curran, Kenneth John, and Somnath Bose

Introduction

Mental health is coming to the forefront of healthcare in modern times. With more attention and research around the topic, there is an enhanced appreciation for the prevalence of psychiatric disease in the general population [1] as well as the intensive care unit (ICU) population. The role of mental health in both the development of and the recovery from severe illness has been acknowledged for many years. It was apparent in the 1970s that patients who required psychiatric consultation were more critically ill than the average ICU patient, having prolonged ICU stays, a more frequent need for mechanical ventilation, and higher mortality rates [2]. The COVID epidemic, starting in 2020, further highlighted this interplay of critical illness and mental health, with larger and younger populations requiring acute medical care and prolonged hospitalization. Yet, this area remains a significantly under-addressed problem due to systemic issues both in medical care outside and inside the hospital. This chapter will review the categories of psychotropic medications commonly encountered in the ICU, broken down by pharmacology, acute intoxication/major side effects, and the challenges with chronic use of these medications. The benefits of continuing these medications during an ICU stay, the role of an ICU as a psychological stressor, and the lasting effects of continuing psychoactive medications past initial hospitalization will also be discussed [3].

S. P. Curran · K. John · S. Bose (✉)
Department of Anesthesia Critical Care and Pain Medicine, Harvard Medical School, Beth Israel Deaconess Medical Center, Boston, MA, USA
e-mail: scurran2@bidmc.harvard.edu; kjohn1@bidmc.harvard.edu; sbose2@bidmc.harvard.edu

K. Karamchandani, J. E. Grant (eds.), *Substance Use Disorders in Adult Critically Ill Patients*, https://doi.org/10.1007/978-3-031-67069-5_9

Benzodiazepines

Pharmacology

The class works by binding to $GABA_A$ receptors. γ-aminobutyric acid (GABA) is a major inhibitory neurotransmitter in the central nervous system and plays an active role in many sedating medications. Benzodiazepines work as positive allosteric modulators and increase the efficacy of GABA neurotransmitters by increasing chloride ion conduction via an increased frequency of channel-opening. This ultimately leads to hyperpolarization of the cell and a reduction in neuronal signaling in the CNS. $GABA_A$ receptors contain 2**α** subunits, 2**β** subunits, and 1γ subunit. Benzodiazepines bind at a specific pocket located at the intersection of the **α** and γ subunits. The benzodiazepine receptor has many subtypes based on the **α** subunit, with the majority of BZD1 receptors found highly concentrated in the cortex, thalamus, and cerebellum.

Benzodiazepines can be administered intramuscularly, intravenously, orally, sublingually, intranasally, or rectally. They are typically highly protein-bound and lipophilic. Intravenous administration usually results in a quick CNS effect with redistribution to adipose tissue. Most benzodiazepines are oxidatively metabolized by the cytochrome P450 enzymes (phase I), conjugated with glucuronide (phase II), and excreted by the kidneys. Some medications will have active metabolites. Diazepam, for example, breaks down into oxazepam, desmethyldiazepam, and temazepam, leading to a longer than expected duration of action and potency of dosing in populations such as the elderly and those with hepatic dysfunction. Additionally, most benzodiazepines and their metabolites are renally excreted, potentially further prolonging the duration of action.

Acute Intoxication/Major Side Effects

At low doses, benzodiazepines exert a calming and anxiolytic effect. Patients also experience anterograde amnesia at varying doses. The effects of benzodiazepines also make them useful as anticonvulsants and muscle relaxants. These features make this class of medications potentially problematic in the elderly population, possibly leading to sources of trauma such as motor vehicle accidents or mechanical falls. In addition to their sedative effects, benzodiazepines can cause confusion, headaches, diarrhea, and nausea/vomiting. This wide range of clinical effects is due to the percentage of GABA receptors activated by a particular dose given. For example, anxiolysis occurs with 20% of receptors bound, whereas hypnosis occurs with at least 60% of receptors activated [4].

Benzodiazepines can unfortunately produce synergistic effects with other common intoxicants, like ethanol, to reduce respiratory drive. Lorazepam and oxazepam additionally interact with the uridine diphosphate glucuronosyltransferases (UGT), which can be upregulated by phenytoin and phenobarbital, medications used for seizures and ethanol withdrawal, respectively.

Misuse of this class is also growing over time, with a five-fold increase in overdose mortality from 1996 to 2013 [5]. Another major concern when using benzodiazepines in the elderly population is the risk of delirium. Special attention should be given when using benzodiazepines, such as Midazolam, as a continuous infusion in elderly patients or those with renal dysfunction. Midazolam has a context-sensitive half-life that leads to the accumulation of active metabolites in these populations of patients [4]. Flumazenil is a specific antidote to benzodiazepine overdose and can rapidly reverse its effects. Though, much like naloxone, a large dose of benzodiazepines may require repeat dosing of flumazenil due to a limited half-life. Seizure is a major concern with withdrawal from high doses or acutely reversing benzodiazepines with flumazenil.

Impact of Chronic Use on Management in the ICU

In the ICU, benzodiazepines are useful for sedation where there is a desire to minimally reduce blood pressure. It is also commonly used to suppress symptoms in alcohol withdrawal, as a muscle relaxant in a patient with spasmodic muscle pain, and to abort seizures in status epilepticus [4]. As mentioned before, using benzodiazepines, particularly for sedation, can lead to delirium in the elderly and critically ill population, so these are best avoided. Additionally, about 5% of the US population is prescribed this medication as a second-line or fast-acting treatment for anxiety [6].

Chronic use may cause tolerance due to the down-regulation of brain receptors for benzodiazepines. Its anxiolytic and euphoric properties have also led to its misuse and physical dependence over time. Stopping these medications when patients have developed dependence can lead to withdrawal, which manifests as anxiety, insomnia, and CNS excitability that can potentially lead to seizures.

Withdrawal from benzodiazepines can appear very similar to that of ethanol withdrawal, leading to an excitable state with tremors, hallucinations, manias, anxiety, and agitation being common [4]. The severity of withdrawal symptoms is based on the dose and frequency of intake of the medication prior to its cessation, with higher chronic doses leading to more profound withdrawal symptoms. There have been many proposed ways to treat withdrawal from benzodiazepines, including beta-blockers (propranolol), or alpha 2 agonists (clonidine, dexmedetomidine), anticonvulsants (valproic acid, lamotrigine, carbamazepine, phenobarbital), progesterone, baclofen, and trazodone—all with mixed results and no significant advantage to benzodiazepine therapy. The current recommendation is to switch from short-acting to long-acting agents, such as Clonazepam, and taper the dose down as an outpatient. Due to its similarity to ethanol, CIWA scoring can be used effectively to monitor and treat benzodiazepine withdrawal.

Selective Serotonin Reuptake Inhibitors/Selective Norepinephrine Reuptake Inhibitors

Pharmacology

As the names describe, reuptake inhibitors work to increase the overall amount of neurotransmitter activity in the synaptic cleft of neurons by blocking their reabsorption into the presynaptic neuron. Serotonin and Norepinephrine Reuptake Inhibitors (SSRIs and SNRIs) therefore, unsurprisingly, work to increase the overall amount of serotonin and norepinephrine in the synaptic cleft. They are both primarily used to treat depression as a first-line medication. In addition to depression, these medications are also used to treat conditions such as fibromyalgia, bipolar disorder, anxiety, and other related conditions [4]. Nearly 17% of patients admitted to the ICU are using an SSRI or SNRI as outpatient medications.

Acute Intoxication/Major Side Effects

SSRIs and SNRIs have relatively fewer side effects compared with older, similar medications; however, there are still a few rare but possible negative effects to be aware of. The first is QT prolongation, which can lead to fatal arrhythmias. This is uncommon and may only be a risk factor in overdose for a couple of the SSRIs and SNRIs, but it has been reported in some case reports. The second potential problem in overdose is serotonin syndrome, which results from excessive activation of postsynaptic serotonin receptors [4]. Serotonin syndrome is also a rare phenomenon. It may present with altered mental status, neuromuscular irritability, and autonomic instability. The most severe reactions occur when multiple medications lead to an increase in serotonin activity. Common medications to be cautious of when utilizing SSRIs or SNRIs include linezolid, meperidine, tramadol, and dextromethorphan [4].

There are a few other infrequent adverse drug reactions to be aware of as well when using SSRIs and SNRIs in the ICU. One is the risk of bleeding due to inhibition of platelet function from serotonin activity. This is more pronounced when patients are on anticoagulants such as aspirin or warfarin. Another effect is an increased risk in vasospasm following an aneurysmal subarachnoid hemorrhage. Lastly, these medications can lead to drug fevers [4].

Impact of Chronic Use on Management in the ICU

In the ICU, SSRIs can be used to supplement or wean off IV sedation medications. They are often limited by their oral formulations, requiring good gastrointestinal tract access. Discontinuation of these medications for patients in the ICU without enteral access can also put a patient at risk of withdrawal, worsen their underlying mental illness, and complicate their overall critical illness [3, 4].

Norepinephrine/Dopamine Reuptake Inhibitors

Pharmacology

Another category whose name describes its action is the Norepinephrine/Dopamine Reuptake Inhibitors (NDRIs), though the exact mechanism of this action is not fully understood. The primary drug of this class is bupropion (Wellbutrin), a commonly used antidepressant and smoking cessation aid. It has three major metabolites as well, all of which have strong noradrenergic activity, which leads to another common off-label use for weight loss [7].

Acute Intoxication/Major Side Effects

Though not commonly started during ICU care, an overdose of NDRIs may present with symptoms as simple as agitation and tachycardia and progress to severe symptoms such as QRS/QT prolongation and seizures. No specific antidote exists for bupropion, and supportive care consists of seizure control and cardiopulmonary support, both of which can necessitate an ICU admission. Though less severe, this category of medication can also cause agitation, constipation, insomnia, and hypertension.

Impact of Chronic Use on Management in the ICU

Though rarely used in an ICU setting, bupropion is a commonly prescribed medication. Although it is unlikely to result in withdrawal symptoms if stopped abruptly, few studies have examined the sudden withdrawal of it in detail. Generally, symptoms related to a rebound of the treated ailment are associated with the withdrawal of the medication, often anxiety, agitation, and insomnia [3].

Monoamine Oxidase Inhibitors

Pharmacology

The mechanism of action of Monoamine Oxidase Inhibitors (MAOI)s is to prevent the degradation of many of the neurotransmitters mentioned so far in the description of other psychoactive medications. Unfortunately, this also means it can interact and interfere with their mechanisms as well. Currently, this category of medications is primarily used to treat resistant and atypical major depressive disorder (MDD), as well as being tested in the management of early Parkinson's disease. The most prescribed member of this category is selegiline, typically as a transdermal patch, which, at lower doses, reduces the drug-food interactions of this class. Notably, many members of this category of medication are irreversible inhibitors whose effects may last weeks.

Acute Intoxication/Major Side Effects

One of the oldest categories of antidepressant medications, MAOIs are often used less frequently due to their broad interactions with both other antidepressants and foods. Cheese and other tyramine-containing foods can trigger severe hypertensive crises when consumed while on MAOIs [8]. Further, SSRIs and MAOIs interact particularly poorly and can lead to the development of Serotonin syndrome. MAOIs also have a low therapeutic index, which can easily lead to overdose with symptoms of agitation, anxiety, flushing, sweating, diplopia, and fever. Severe overdoses can lead to seizures, confusion, hallucinations, altered mental status, and coma.

Impact of Chronic Use on Management in the ICU

Withdrawal from MAOIs can be similar to withdrawal from other antidepressants with anxiety, agitation, and insomnia. While not typically started in the ICU, this category of drugs can potentially interfere with many of the medications used in an ICU setting, particularly SSRIs that may be used for sedation. Interdisciplinary aid with psychiatric and potentially pharmacy consultations is highly encouraged.

Tricyclic Antipsychotics

Pharmacology

Originally developed in the 1950s, Tricyclic Antipsychotics (TCAs) are now considered second-line treatments for depression, insomnia, obsessive-compulsive disorder, and pain disorders like diabetic neuropathy and fibromyalgia. This category is named for its chemical structure of three rings that allow it to interfere with the reuptake transporters of five different neurotransmitters. It is very important to confirm a patient's medication history before starting an SSRI in the ICU for this reason [9].

Acute Intoxication/Major Side Effects

Due to their broad side effects, they are generally prescribed less frequently than SSRIs or SNRIs. They may produce QTc prolongation. Overdose of TCAs as part of a suicide attempt is not uncommon and requires management of several pathways of toxicity: lidocaine for cardiac effects, benzodiazepines for seizures, fluids and pressors for hypotension from adrenergic blockade, and the previously mentioned serotonin syndrome. Active charcoal and other means for removing TCAs before they can be absorbed is a major part of treatment as well.

Impact of Chronic Use on Management in the ICU

Withdrawal is relatively minor compared with most psychoactive medications, consisting primarily of agitation, headaches, and GI hyperactivity. However, there can also be a rebound of the ailments that they are prescribed to treat, which can confound differential diagnoses.

Antipsychotics

Pharmacology

Antipsychotics can be broken down into two broad categories: 1st generation (typical antipsychotics) and 2nd generation (atypical antipsychotics). These medications are typically used to treat schizophrenia and other psychotic disorders but have been shown to be effective in treating acute agitation and delirium in the ICU. Typical antipsychotics work primarily by dopamine (D2) receptor activation. They also have noradrenergic, cholinergic, and histamine-blocking actions. Atypical antipsychotics work as both dopamine and serotonin receptor agonists. The common typical antipsychotic used in the ICU includes haloperidol, and the common atypical antipsychotics include olanzapine and quetiapine.

Acute Intoxication/Major Side Effects

The effect on D2-receptors is what leads to extrapyramidal symptoms (EPS) seen with medications such as haloperidol [4]. EPS symptoms can present as acute dystonia (more common in young males), akathisia, parkinsonism (more common in females), tremors, or tardive dyskinesia. There is also a higher risk of torsades de pointes with typical antipsychotics, especially in the setting of hypokalemia and hypomagnesemia [4].

Neuroleptic malignant syndrome is a rare but fatal adverse effect that can occur with typical antipsychotics. Symptoms can present over the course of 24–72 hours with fevers, severe muscular rigidity, confusion, agitation, leukocytosis, elevated creatinine phosphokinase concentrations, elevated liver enzymes, myoglobinuria, and acute renal failure. Treatment includes stopping the antipsychotic and initiating dantrolene therapy, along with intravenous hydration, external cooling, and close monitoring of vital signs and electrolytes.

There are far fewer incidences of EPS with this new generation of antipsychotics. However, there are other side effects to be aware of, such as QT prolongation, drowsiness, ventricular tachycardia, fever, and neutropenia [4]. Atypical antipsychotics are also more expensive than typical antipsychotics and, therefore, less commonly prescribed.

Impact of Chronic Use on Management in the ICU

Withdrawal from antipsychotic medications can vary in presentation and affect multiple organ systems. Symptoms can appear like the beginning of a psychotic relapse, with features like agitation and insomnia. Also common are hypoactivity, hyperkinesia with involuntary, movements and ataxia. The treatment of choice is to restart the patient's home medication and, if necessary, initiate a slow taper to find the appropriate dosing for the patient.

Stimulants

Stimulants are a broad category of medications seeing more and more use in the general population, both for treatment of conditions such as attention-deficit hyperactivity disorder (ADHD) or narcolepsy. The peak age for prescribing stimulants to a patient for the diagnosis of ADHD is between 5 and 11 years [10]. These medications are prescribed to males 2.5 times more often than females. However, there is growing concern of underdiagnosis and treatment of ADHD in girls during their childhood [11]. Although there has been a persistent concern regarding over-prescribing stimulants, surveys show that we are likely under-treating the diagnosis, with the prevalence of ADHD outweighing the percentage of children receiving treatment, 8.6% versus 4.6%, respectively [12].

The prevalence of ADHD in adults is reduced to 2.5%. The drop off in prescription of stimulants as people age into adulthood correlates with a reduction in impulsivity and hyperactivity for most people [13]. The first-line stimulants used for ADHD are methylphenidate and amphetamine. Both medications reduce the reuptake of norepinephrine and dopamine in the brain regions of the cortex and striatum, influencing executive and attentional function [14]. These medications are made in both long- and short-acting formularies, allowing for tailored prescribing to a patient's lifestyle needs or preferences. Both medications also come with a wide variety of adverse effects, such as decreased appetite, sleep disturbances, increased blood pressure and pulse, headaches, irritability, and stomach pain [15]. Most often, these symptoms are mild in nature and generally tolerated by patients.

Impact of Chronic Use on Management in the ICU

Depending on the clinical scenario, it may or may not be appropriate to restart these medications in an ICU setting. Withdrawal from stimulants like methylphenidate is not commonly described outside of case reports that describe rare signs and symptoms. More commonly, one may see patients requesting, or potentially craving, the continuation of their home dose of the medication to prevent the return of their symptoms [16].

Benefits of Restarting Home Psychoactive Medications

In a 2018 national survey of over 36,000 US adults, Hasin and colleagues found that the 12-month and lifetime prevalences of MDD were 10.4% and 20.6%, respectively. A majority of these individuals had moderate or severe MDD, with three-quarters of cases involving anxiety. Not only has there been a rise in diagnosis over the years, but 70% of lifetime MDD patients received some type of treatment to combat the illness [17].

The use of psychotropic medications for adults in the US has increased from the late 1980s to the present time. Since that time, there has been a three-fold increase in antidepressant use, specifically. When looking at a population of children and young adults, antidepressant use increases with age, with the highest use found in young adults aged 24 years. Antipsychotics were the least prescribed psychotropic medications versus antidepressants and stimulants [18].

Recognizing that many patients admitted to the ICU are taking psychoactive medications at home is only half the battle for this topic. The second half is restarting their home medications to reduce the amount of discontinuous time from their last dose. Abrupt discontinuation of home psychotropic medications is common among critically ill patients but may precipitate clinically significant withdrawal. About half of patients admitted to the ICU will have interruptions to their home psychotropic medications for at least 24 hours [19]. This can happen due to a lack of administration access (i.e., no enteral access) while patients are critically ill, as well as a gap in time from their admission to when a comprehensive home medication reconciliation is done. In this same population of ICU patients, 16% of patients will ultimately not have their medications restarted during their admission. Unfortunately for these patients, they are more likely to have a longer ICU length of stay and greater incidence of ICU delirium with greater acute antipsychotic use [19, 20]. When restarting home psychoactive medications, patients in the ICU also have a lower RASS-score, requiring less sedation and leading to less sedation-related delirium [21].

As we reviewed in the previous section, withdrawal symptoms of the typical psychoactive medications can lead to symptoms severe enough to warrant an ICU admission. Holding home medication can inadvertently lead to these withdrawal symptoms. By getting a patient back to their home regimen of medications, we ensure that they are on a stable dose prior to discharge. As we will cover in the next section, the ICU environment itself is a major source of psychiatric stress, so controlling patients with preexisting psychiatric disorders with their home medications is prudent for their overall well-being and recovering from critical illness.

The Role of the ICU as a Psychiatric Stressor

Although patients may come to the ICU with pre-existing psychiatric disease, there is also a significant-sized population of patients who will be discharged after an admission to the ICU with a long-lasting psychiatric condition. Psychiatric symptoms and disorders affect about 15–35% of patients' months after ICU discharge [22]. Major psychiatric illnesses that have been noted to persist months after an ICU admission include anxiety, depression, and PTSD [23, 24]. These patients, unfortunately, are found to have a worse health-related quality of life (HRQoL) versus patients without psychiatric disorders. In fact, the more psychiatric syndromes that a patient develops in the time after their time in the ICU, the worse their HRQoL scores are [23].

There are specific stressors in the ICU that function as psychiatric stressors that can lead to agitation or delirium and result in prescribing psychotropic medications to control symptoms. A large contributor to psychiatric symptoms is the lack of a regular sleep cycle. Sleep in the ICU is often disrupted by frequent evaluations, examinations, and procedures with the urgency to be done overnight. Delirium can also develop in patients who are sedated for a prolonged period. Daily wakening episodes with a break from sedation help reduce the risk for psychiatric complications.

Post-Intensive Care Syndrome (PICS) is defined by the Society of Critical Care Medicine as a constellation of new or worsened physical and psychological health problems stemming from and remaining after a critical illness. Anxiety, depression, memory issues, and PTSD are commonly seen. Screening for symptoms of post-traumatic stress, anxiety, and depression at one week from ICU discharge can correlate with a risk of having PICS at three months post admission to the ICU [25]. It is estimated that around 14% of critically ill patients will continue to have PICS, with a greater risk associated with experiencing frightening situations in the ICU, baseline elevated pain scores, the presence of anxiety or depression, and poor sleep quality months after discharge [26].

Treatment of PICS is difficult, and the bulk of efforts are currently focused on prevention during the ICU stay. A major component of this is providing the patient with normalizing behaviors while still in the ICU, such as ICU diaries, maintaining day-wake cycles, and regular re-orientation. Utilizing clinical psychologist support can lead to lower rates of anxiety and depression as well as risk for PTSD after an ICU admission. This also led to fewer patients requiring psychiatric medications at 12 months [27]. The use of psychoactive medications is recommended and sometimes even required during this process, but an emphasis is placed on avoiding oversedation. It is, however, not uncommon to see the doses of psychoactive medications maintained after transfer from the ICU and even from the hospital without adjustment [28, 29]. In the last section of this chapter, we review the risks and benefits of continuing psychiatric medications after ICU discharge.

Effects of Continuing Psychiatric Medications After ICU Recovery

In a large study looking at nearly 4000 ICU admissions over seven years, 8% of patients were started on new antipsychotic medications [30]. Interestingly, these new prescriptions do not end after ICU discharge. At least half to three-quarters of ICU patients who started new antipsychotic medications continued these medications after being discharged from the ICU [31]. The momentum continues as one-third of these patients will continue their antipsychotics after discharge from the hospital [28, 30]. This trend is concerning for multiple reasons. When treating teams were asked by pharmacists why their patients were on antipsychotics after ICU discharge, half of the respondents were unsure or had an incorrect indication for the treatment [28]. Another concerning detail is that patients who continued antipsychotics as outpatients had increased odds of being co-prescribed opiates and/or benzodiazepines, leading to potential polypharmacy complications [32]. One reassuring finding is that new antipsychotic prescriptions were not associated with increased health resource utilization (i.e., 72-hour ICU readmission and 30-day emergency room visitation or hospitalization) [32].

Part of the issue seems to stem from a lack of documentation and handoff between providers on why a medication was started, leading to a reluctance to discontinue it. Many of the medications utilized have side effects relating to sedation, which adds to the problems of oversedation and disorientation caused by the time in the ICU. SSRIs are a major culprit in this due to the fact that they are prescribed to help with ventilator tolerance. However, after discharge, the use of these medications is not associated with improvements in mortality or readmission; however, the long-term implications on persistent use or abuse remain unclear [32].

These medications also have the potential to negatively affect patients after they are discharged from the hospital. For example, patients who continued to take SNRIs or a combination of psychiatric medications had a lower health-related quality of life [33]. Other medications are hepatotoxic, lead to thrombocytopenia, falls from dizziness, or even simply persistent sedation. Separating these from their direct effects on the patient, the added burden of additional medical care, disruptions to daily life, and interruptions to recovery can lead to poor outcomes. As recovery from PICS emphasizes a return to normalization, these persistent reminders can greatly limit progress.

Geriatric populations are especially vulnerable to this iatrogenic, somewhat modifiable phenomenon. They are known to experience higher rates of delirium during hospital stays, often in turn leading to the prescription of psychoactive medications. Several studies have found an association in all-cause mortality among the older population with multiple categories with these prescriptions [34].

An ICU stay is a traumatic event. Compromises are often made on the side of patient survival over patient comfort. While this makes sense at the time, the balance changes as the patient's general health recovers. Many patients do require some type of psychoactive medication to help them through recovery, but many others will have their recovery delayed by medications they no longer need [35]. Reassessment by psychiatry consultants at multiple points during and after the hospital stay is necessary to assess this, as multiple studies have shown. Several efforts are underway to better require these reassessments before discharge using the electronic health records [36] and active reconciliation tools, but awareness of the long-term consequences of medications originally prescribed for short-term indications needs further emphasis.

References

1. Paulose-Ram R, Safran MA, et al. Trends in psychotropic medication use among US adults. Pharmacoepidemiol Drug Saf. 2007;16(5):560–70. https://doi.org/10.1002/pds.1367.
2. Hale M, Koss N, et al. Psychiatric complications in a surgical ICU. Critical Care Med. 1977;5(4):199–203.
3. Katzung BG, Masters SB, Trevor AJ. Basic and clinical pharmacology. McGraw Hill. 11th Edition. Copyright 2009.
4. Shafiekhani M, Mirjalili M, Vazin A. Psychotropic drug therapy in patients in the intensive care unit – usage, adverse effects, and drug interactions: a review. Ther Clin Risk Manag. 2018;28(14):1799–812. https://doi.org/10.2147/TCRM.S176079. PMID: 30319262; PMCID: PMC6168070
5. Bachhuber MA, Hennessy S, Cunningham CO, et al. Increasing Benzodiazepine prescriptions and overdose mortality in the United States, 1996–2013. Am J Public Health. 2016;106:686–8.
6. Maust DT, Lin LA, Blow FC. Benzodiazepine use and misuse among adults in the United States. Psychiatr Serv. 2019;70(2):97-106. https://doi.org/10.1176/appi.ps.201800321. Epub 2018 Dec 17. PMID: 30554562; PMCID: PMC6358464.
7. Alberter AA, Chambers AJ, Wills BK. Bupropion toxicity. StatPearls [Internet]. StatPearls Publishing, 2022. Updated December 12, 2022.
8. Laban TS, Saadabadi A. Monoamine oxidase inhibitors (MAOI). StatPearls [Internet]. StatPearls Publishing, 2022. Updated July 17 2023.
9. Moraczewski J,Aedma KK. Tricyclic antidepressants. StatPearls [Internet]. StatPearls Publishing, 2022. Updated August 17 2023.
10. Kessler RC, Amminger GP, et al. Age of onset of mental disorders: a review of recent literature. Curr Opin Psychiatry. 2007;20:359–64.
11. Quinn P, Madhoo M. A review of attention-deficit/hyperactivity disorder in women and girls: uncovering this hidden diagnosis. Primary Care Companion CNS Disord. 2014; 16:PCC.13r01596.
12. Olfson M, He JP, Merikangas KR. Psychotropic medication treatment of adolescents: results from the national comorbidity survey-adolescent supplement. J Am Acad Child Adolesc Psychiatry. 2013;52:378–88.
13. Hollbrook JR, Cuffe SP, et al. Persistence of parent-reported ADHD symptoms from childhood through adolescence in a community sample. J Atten Disord. 2016;20:11–20.
14. Faraone S. The pharmacology of Amphetamine and Methylphenidate: relevance to the neurobiology of attention-deficit/hyperactivity disorder and other psychiatric comorbidities. Neurosci Biobehav Rev. 2018;87:255–70.
15. Mechler K, Banaschewski T, Hohmann S, Hage A. Evidence-based pharmacological treatment options for ADHD in children and adolescents. Pharmacol Therapeut. 2022; 230.
16. Spiller HA, Hays HL, Aleguas A Jr. Overdose of drugs for attention-deficit hyperactivity disorder: clinical presentation, mechanisms of toxicity, and management. CNS Drugs. 2013;27:531–43.
17. Hasin DS, Sarvet AL, Meyers JL, et al. Epidemiology of adult DSM-5 major depressive disorder and its specifiers in the United States. JAMA Psychiat. 2018;75(4):336–46. https://doi.org/10.1001/jamapsychiatry.2017.4602.
18. Sultan RS, Correll CU, Schoenbaum M, King M, Walkup JT, Olfson M. National patterns of commonly prescribed psychotropic medications to young people. J Child Adolesc Psychopharmacol. 2018;28(3):158–65. https://doi.org/10.1089/cap.2017.0077. Epub 2018 Jan 29. PMID: 29376743; PMCID: PMC5905871
19. Atherton J, Abdrabbo M, Kassab H. Impact of abrupt interruption of home psychotropic medications at ICU admission. J Pharm Technol 2023;39(4). https://doi.org/10.1177/87551225231182286

20. Li M, Chang MH, et al. Impact of early home psychotropic medication reinitiation on surrogate measures of intensive care unit delirium. Mental Health Clin. 2019;9(4):263–8. https://doi.org/10.9740/mhc.2019.07.263.
21. La MK, Thompson Bastin ML, et al. Impact of restarting home neuropsychiatric medications on sedation outcomes in medical intensive care unit patients. J Crit Care. 2018;43:102–7.
22. Weinert C. Epidemiology and treatment of psychiatric conditions that develop after critical illness. Curr Opin Crit Care. 2005;11(4):376–80. https://doi.org/10.1097/01.ccx.0000168529.23078.64.
23. Teixeira C, Rosa RG, et al. The burden of mental illness among survivors of critical care – risk factors and impact on quality of life: a multicenter prospective cohort study. CHEST. 2021;160(1):157–64. https://doi.org/10.1016/j.chest.2021.02.034.
24. Janssen DGA, Jonker J, van Dijk D, Heerdink ER, Egberts TCG, Slooter AJC. Psychotropic medication use in former ICU patients with mental health problems: a prospective observational follow-up study. J Crit Care. 2020;59:112–7. https://doi.org/10.1016/j.jcrc.2020.06.002. Epub 2020 Jun 9
25. Milton A, Bruck E, et al. Early psychological screening of intensive unit survivors: a prospective cohort study. Crit Care. 2017;21:273.
26. Elliot R, McKinley S, et al. Posttraumatic stress symtoms in intensive care patients: an exploration of associated factors. Rehab Psychol. 2016;61(2):141–50.
27. Peris A, Bonizzoli M, Iozzelli D, Migliaccio ML, Zagli G, Bacchereti A, Debolini M, Vannini E, Solaro M, Balzi I, Bendoni E, Bacchi I, Trevisan M, Giovannini V, Belloni L. Early intra-intensive care unit psychological intervention promotes recovery from post traumatic stress disorders, anxiety and depression symptoms in critically ill patients. Crit Care. 2011;15(1):R41. https://doi.org/10.1186/cc10003. Epub 2011 Jan 27. Erratum in: Crit Care. 2011;15(2):418. Trevisan, Monica [added]. PMID: 21272307; PMCID: PMC3221970.
28. Kovacic NL, Gagnon DJ, Fraser GL. An analysis of psychoactive medications initiated in the ICU but continued beyond discharge: a pilot study of stewardship. J Pharm Pract. 2019;33(6) https://doi.org/10.1177/0897190019830518.
29. Short A, McPeake J, Andonovic M, et al. Medication-related problems in critical care survivors: a systematic review. Eur J Hosp Pharm. 2023;30:250–6.
30. Marshall J, Herzig SJ, et al. Antipsychotic utilization in the intensive care unit and in transitions of care. J Crit Care. 2016;33(1):119–24. https://doi.org/10.1016/j.jcrc.2015.12.01.
31. Jasiak KD, Middleton EA, et al. Evaluation of discontinuation of atypical antipsychotics prescribed for ICU delirium. J Pharm Pract. 2012;26(3) https://doi.org/10.1177/0897190012465987.
32. Jaworska N, et al. Impacts of antipsychotic medication prescribing practices in critically ill adult patients on health resource utilization and new psychoactive medication prescriptions. PLoS One. 2023;18(6):e0287929.
33. Alfaifi AA, Althemery AU. Sociodemographic characteristics and health-related quality of life of individuals undergoing antidepressant therapy. Sci Rep. 2022;12:17518. https://doi.org/10.1038/s41598-022-22164-6.
34. Du Y, Wolf IK, Busch MA, Knopf H. Associations between the use of specific psychotropic drugs and all-cause mortality among older adults in Germany: results of the mortality follow-up of the German National Health Interview and Examination Survey 1998. PLoS One. 2019;14(1):e0210695.
35. Olafson K, et al. The 5-year pre-and post-hospitalization treated prevalence of mental disorders and psychotropic medication use in critically ill patients: a Canadian population-based study. Intensive Care Med. 2021;47:1450–61.
36. Flaws D, et al. A protocol for a pilot randomised controlled trial of an Early Psychiatric Assessment, Referral, and Intervention Study (EPARIS) for intensive care patients. PLoS One. 2023;18(6):e0287470.

Chapter 10
Treatment of Substance Use Disorders in Post-ICU Settings

Stephen V. Marcoux

Patients with substance use disorders (SUDs) present in multiple settings within a spectrum of acute intoxication, withdrawal, a period of sobriety, or relapse. After intensive care treatment, while patients may be stabilized from intoxication or severe withdrawal, the ongoing management of the SUD requires continued observation and treatment of withdrawal symptoms and immediate discussion and intervention regarding therapeutic and pharmacotherapy options for abstinence and treatment management.

To affirm prior chapters' discussion, substance abuse, simply put, involves improper use of a substance, which can lead to negative physical or psychological health effects. Substance dependence, escalating from abuse, involves not only negative impacts on physical and psychological health but also a physiological reliance on a substance. With the publication of the updated Diagnostic and Statistical Manual of Mental Disorders, fifth edition, the term substance use disorder was introduced, with specifiers of mild, moderate, and severe, encompassing prior abuse and dependence classifications [1]. A SUD involves clearly defined symptoms, both biological and psychosocial, as a consequence of substance use, leading to significant impairment in components of daily functioning.

The development of a SUD involves both psychological and biological factors. From a neurobiological perspective, addiction manifestation is associated with feedback-reward circuitry. The reward circuitry involves multiple corticostriatal pathways linking the prefrontal cortex, anterior cingulate cortex, and orbitofrontal cortex (all involved in executive functioning—critical thinking/decision making, impulse control, anticipation, etc.) to the ventral tegmental area, nucleus accumbens (providing reward neurotransmitter release), and amygdala (emotional center). The

S. V. Marcoux (✉)
Department of Psychiatry and Behavioral Neuroscience, University of Chicago Medical Center, Chicago, IL, USA
e-mail: Stephen.Marcoux@uchicagomedicine.org

K. Karamchandani, J. E. Grant (eds.), *Substance Use Disorders in Adult Critically Ill Patients*, https://doi.org/10.1007/978-3-031-67069-5_10

release of dopamine after a stimulus can produce positive emotions (euphoria and sense of reward), with the amount and frequency of dopamine release (and receptor sensitization) impacting conditioning to a stimulus and motivation to continue the stimulus. This conditioning process involves neuroadaptation, leading to an intense desire for a substance. This intense desire for the substance, coupled with the negative impact of stopping the substance (due to receptor downregulation and desensitization), provides continued feedback loops of ongoing substance use, eventually leading to tolerance and physiological dependence on the substance. The substances discussed in this chapter either have a direct or indirect impact on dopamine release and the subsequent reward circuitry feedback loop [2–4].

This chapter will discuss the continued management of patients with a SUD after stabilization in the intensive care unit (ICU). The substances that will be discussed are organized by class and chosen due to their prevalence in hospital settings to provide realistic and practical guidance on treatment management after stabilization in the ICU.

Substance Use Disorder Evaluation and Treatment

Given the prevalence of SUDs in hospitalized patients, completion of a basic substance use history with associated laboratory evaluation, initiation of appropriate substance withdrawal treatment, and introducing prevention and/or maintenance measures are vital to decreasing patient morbidity.

Obtaining a substance use history greatly assists with assessing the risk of withdrawal from a substance, evaluating the severity of the substance use disorder, and guiding the level of intervention needed for the management of the SUD. The diagnosis of a SUD requires an evaluation of 12 separate biological or psychological effects from the problematic pattern of substance use and leading to significant impairment or distress over a one-year period. Examples of such effects of substance use include: increasing the amount of the substance for desired effect, often greater than intended amount of the substance is used, inability to cut down use of the substance, a great deal of time is spent in activities necessary to obtain or recover from the substance effects, craving or strong desire to use the substance, recurrent use resulting in failure to fulfill work/home obligations, continued use despite interpersonal problems, continued use despite medical or psychological problems worsened by the substance, substance use in situations that are hazardous, reduction in other activities due to substance use, and/or withdrawal symptoms after substance cessation[1].

A substance use history in a hospital setting should involve, at a minimum, assessing the amount, frequency, route of administration, duration of use, history of withdrawal, and most recent amount and timing of the last use for each substance. Other helpful data include first use, pattern and circumstances surrounding use, prior substance rehabilitation, efforts to stop substance use, and the legal/social impact of substance use. Should a patient present intoxicated or unable to provide a substance use history, collateral information from friends or family is recommended to better assist with treatment [5].

Types of substances that should be assessed in a thorough substance use evaluation include alcohol, benzodiazepines (sedatives/anxiolytics/hypnotics), cannabis, hallucinogens, opioids, stimulants, and tobacco (nicotine products). A full medical history (to include psychiatric symptoms, diagnoses, and treatment) and medication reconciliation are also essential to assess the substance use's impact on general medical conditions and the interactions of medications with an individual's substance use.

1. Alcohol withdrawal and alcohol use disorder

After stabilization in the intensive care unit, patients with alcohol withdrawal may continue to require observation and management. Patients with severe alcohol use disorder may manifest alcohol withdrawal symptoms more than 72 hours after alcohol cessation and present initially with acute delirium or hallucinations more rapidly than other patients. Patients intubated with sedating agents may have delayed and prolonged withdrawal symptoms post-extubation, as non-benzodiazepine or barbiturate sedating agents may mask autonomic and clinical signs of withdrawal, leading to rebound withdrawal presentations when these agents are discontinued.

In evaluating patients at risk of withdrawal and possible alcohol use disorder after ICU stabilization, consideration of multiple laboratory studies is indicated. Awareness of the patient's initial admission blood ethanol level and severity of intoxication impairment is helpful to assess the patient's level of toleration of alcohol. Complete Blood Count (CBC) values can indicate chronic use of alcohol, specifically macrocytic anemia, due to bone marrow suppression [6]. Vitamin B12, Thiamine, Folate, Vitamin D, and Vitamin A (amongst others) deficiencies can occur due to poor nutrition and gastrointestinal malabsorption from chronic alcohol use [7]. In severe alcohol use disorder, a lower platelet count, elevated bilirubin, lower albumin, and significantly elevated liver enzymes can indicate liver dysfunction. Gamma glutamyl transferase, carbohydrate-deficient transferrin, phosphatidyl ethanol, and ethyl glucuronide are biomarkers that can be useful to detect chronic alcohol use. Phosphatidyl ethanol (Peth) and ethyl glucuronide are the most sensitive and specific for alcohol use and are used primarily in substance use treatment centers, liver transplant programs, and forensic cases [8]. In evaluating laboratory data and obtaining a substance use history, the determination of the level of acute withdrawal treatment can be identified, with subsequent discussion of preventative measures of continued substance use.

Initial symptom monitoring is indicated for patients who have either known heavy alcohol use, history of alcohol withdrawal, abnormal lab values indicating possible heavy alcohol use, and/or suspicion of recent heavy alcohol use in the context of medical presentation/medical co-morbidities (liver failure, cardiomyopathy, etc.). The Clinical Institute Withdrawal Assessment of Alcohol Scale (CIWA-Ar) is an evidence-based tool for evaluating symptoms of alcohol withdrawal, which include anxiety, agitation, auditory disturbances, visual disturbances, tactile disturbances, clouding of sensorium, tremor, paroxysmal sweats, headaches, and nausea/vomiting [9].

Alcohol withdrawal symptom manifestation typically occurs within 6–12 hours after the cessation of alcohol. Initial withdrawal symptoms involve tremor, nausea/vomiting, headache, hypertension, sweating, tachycardia, anxiety, and insomnia. Hallucinations can typically occur 12–24 hours after alcohol cessation, with seizures occurring 24–48 hours after alcohol cessation. Alcohol withdrawal delirium, which includes disorientation, hallucinations, sweating, tremor, and agitation, occurs typically 48–72 hours after alcohol cessation. However, the clinical course can vary significantly by medical conditions, chronic alcohol use history, etc., with withdrawal symptoms sometimes manifesting >72 hours after last alcohol consumption and thus may occur after ICU stabilization [2, 10, 11]. As in the ICU, the treatment for alcohol withdrawal involves careful monitoring of withdrawal symptoms, utilizing vital sign measurements and CIWA-Ar scoring, supportive nutritional supplementation (magnesium and/or phosphorus as clinically indicated, thiamine, folate), intravenous (IV) hydration, and administering benzodiazepines (or alternative agents if benzodiazepines contraindicated or refractory withdrawal symptoms) until withdrawal symptoms subside. Once withdrawal symptoms have decreased and stabilized, a slow taper of the benzodiazepine should occur, typically a reduction in dosage by roughly 25% every 3–5 days in the hospital setting. It is recommended to continue CIWA-Ar scale monitoring throughout front-loading, fixed dosing administration, and tapering to ensure withdrawal symptoms are adequately controlled. Frequent monitoring of vital signs, particularly oxygen saturation/respirations should also occur given persistent benzodiazepine utilization [5, 12, 13].

Supportive treatment, which should include intravenous (IV) hydration, IV/PO Thiamine, and other vitamin and electrolyte supplementation, should occur concurrently during alcohol withdrawal treatment. Non-pharmacological interventions should include frequent re-orientation, frequent vital sign observations, and minimally stimulating environments. If alcohol withdrawal hallucinations and agitation are severe, adjunctive antipsychotic use (second-generation atypical antipsychotics such as Quetiapine) can be utilized in conjunction with benzodiazepines [5]. If autonomic hyperactivity is not controlled by benzodiazepines, clonidine can be used adjunctly. If tachycardia or hypertension is not adequately controlled by benzodiazepines, beta blockers can be used adjunctly.

The management of an alcohol use disorder relies on pharmacological and therapeutic interventions. Patients admitted to the hospital with either concern for alcohol use disorder or admitted for/experienced alcohol withdrawal and not currently in withdrawal should be assessed for interest in alcohol cessation and defined treatment goals. Education regarding the risks of continued alcohol use on physical and mental health should be completed. If the patient meets criteria for alcohol use disorder, recommendations for both non-pharmacological (rehabilitation/therapy) and pharmacological treatment should be advised and documented; however, participation in these recommendations is voluntary. Within a medical hospital, consultation with case managers, social workers, and, if available, substance use counselors, are recommended to discuss options with the patient and provide local resources, while also assisting with scheduling appts and/or program enrollment [2, 10, 13, 14].

Pharmacotherapy for alcohol use disorder primarily targets craving/desire to use alcohol. These medications should be considered for initiation after the patient has resolved alcohol withdrawal symptoms within the hospital setting. Three medications are FDA-approved for treating alcohol use disorder: Naltrexone, Acamprosate, and Disulfiram. Naltrexone and Acamprosate are preferred options based on clinical evidence and their side effect/safety profile. Disulfiram has historically been used; however, clinical evidence of effectiveness is mixed with the risk of adverse reactions if used with alcohol [15].

2. Benzodiazepine withdrawal and sedative/hypnotic/anxiolytic use disorder

After stabilization in the ICU, benzodiazepine withdrawal will likely require ongoing observation and management. Benzodiazepine withdrawal can be life-threatening if not identified, monitored, and treated. The timing and severity of withdrawal depend on the type of benzodiazepine utilized and the associated half-life. Alprazolam, Temazepam, and Oxazepam have shorter half-lives, and thus withdrawal symptoms can manifest within 24 hours after discontinuation and peak by 48 hours, with withdrawal symptoms persisting up to 2–4 weeks. Longer-acting benzodiazepines like diazepam or chlordiazepoxide can take 5–6 days (some studies, 2–7 days) or longer before the onset of withdrawal symptoms, with withdrawal persisting for 2–8 weeks or more. It remains imperative to obtain an adequate medication reconciliation and substance use history to include frequency, amount, and prolonged use of benzodiazepines to assist in identifying risk factors and the likelihood of severity of benzodiazepine withdrawal. Benzodiazepine withdrawal symptoms include autonomic hyperactivity (sweating, tachycardia), hand tremor, insomnia, nausea/vomiting, transient visual/tactile/auditory hallucinations, psychomotor agitation, anxiety, and grand mal seizures, along with disturbances in mood (dysphoria, irritability, obsessive rumination), photophobia, muscle twitching, and dysesthesia. Mild withdrawal symptoms such as anxiety or insomnia manifest in the first few days, followed by moderate and severe withdrawal symptoms of tremor, nausea/vomiting, sweating, seizures, and psychosis (severe symptoms) from day 2–14 [2, 10, 16–18].

Initial symptom monitoring is indicated for patients who have either known chronic benzodiazepine use (prescribed or not prescribed), history of benzodiazepine or alcohol withdrawal, and positive urine toxicology for benzodiazepines. The Clinical Institute Withdrawal Assessment of Alcohol Scale (CIWA-Ar) is validated only for alcohol withdrawal; however, given the similarity in symptoms and mechanism of withdrawal in comparison to benzodiazepines, it can be utilized to assist with the assessment of withdrawal symptoms. CIWA-Benzodiazepine is a modified CIWA scale utilized for benzodiazepines; however, it is not always available or utilized across all institutions. CIWA-Ar symptoms evaluated include anxiety, agitation, auditory disturbances, visual disturbances, tactile disturbances, clouding of sensorium, tremor, paroxysmal sweats, headaches, and nausea/vomiting, all of which remain notably similar to benzodiazepine withdrawal symptoms [19, 20].

The treatment of benzodiazepine withdrawal on the nursing floor involves the initiation of replacement benzodiazepines to ensure the avoidance of severe withdrawal and instill a safe down-titration of the medication. After completing a clinical evaluation of concurrent medical and psychiatric conditions, obtaining a benzodiazepine use history, evaluating urine toxicology data, along with assessing benzodiazepine withdrawal symptoms, a determination of the typical stabilizing benzodiazepine dose should be obtained. This stabilizing benzodiazepine dose initiation is to treat/resolve benzodiazepine withdrawal utilizing an adequate typical dose the patient had been taking previously. CIWA-Ar, or if available CIWA-Benzodiazepine, monitoring can be helpful to assist with the level of withdrawal and to evaluate use of benzodiazepines over a 24-hour period should there be delays in the initiation of stabilizing and subsequent tapered dose reduction of a benzodiazepine during hospitalization. Mechanistically, longer-acting benzodiazepines are preferable as they lead to less rebound symptoms and less risk for breakthrough anxiety/withdrawal symptoms. However, with hepatic dysfunction, lorazepam remains the optimal option due to less hepatic metabolism and intermediate half-life, and thus would avoid clonazepam, chlordiazepoxide, or diazepam due to primary hepatic metabolism. In renal dysfunction, some research indicates Lorazepam as the most optimal option at lower doses. Once the patient is on a stabilizing benzodiazepine dose and acute withdrawal symptoms have ceased, a methodical reduction in the benzodiazepine is indicated. Dose reduction strategies vary; however, typical toleration involves either 50% dose reduction every week, 10–25% dose reduction every few days, or 25% every one to 2 weeks, depending on the patient.

Alternative treatments for benzodiazepine withdrawal have limited data for efficacy. Propranolol, clonidine, valproate, lamotrigine, carbamazepine, pregabalin, gabapentin, phenobarbital, progesterone, buspirone, paroxetine, baclofen, and trazodone have been proposed with some study; however, all have received either mixed-benefit results, not enough empirical evidence for efficacy, or were not found to be more efficacious than benzodiazepines. Oxcarbazepine and captodiamine have some promising positive studies as benzodiazepine alternatives to manage withdrawal symptoms however data and safety testing is limited. Flumazenil utilization alone and in conjunction with benzodiazepines has been evaluated in several randomized control trials with some benefit noted for withdrawal symptoms vs. placebo and benzodiazepines alone; however, data remains limited and without enough evidence regarding safety (higher seizure risk) and overall efficacy of the intervention [2, 10, 16, 18, 21–24].

Management of sedative/hypnotic/anxiolytic use disorder relies on pharmacological intervention initially to assist with the severity of withdrawal; however, long-term treatment primarily involves therapeutic interventions. There are currently no FDA-approved pharmacological agents for the treatment of sedative/hypnotic/anxiolytic use disorder. Patients admitted to the hospital with either concern for sedative/hypnotic/anxiolytic use and not currently in withdrawal should be assessed for interest in sedative/hypnotic/anxiolytic cessation and defined treatment goals. Not all patients with benzodiazepine or other sedative/hypnotic/anxiolytic withdrawal are abusing these substances, as these medications may be prescribed (for multiple medication conditions) and then subsequently stopped suddenly due to acute medical decompensation or trauma. Careful evaluation of prescribed medications and affirmation of use through pharmacy contact and prescription drug monitoring programs (PDMPs) is helpful to evaluate if prescription abuse has occurred. Patients should also be screened for co-occurring psychiatric conditions, as benzodiazepine utilization may have been initiated for a psychiatric disorder and subsequently transformed into an associated substance use disorder. Education regarding the risks of continued benzodiazepine use on physical and mental health should be completed. Outside of elevated risk for dependence, chronic benzodiazepine use has been found in some studies to increase the risk of cognitive decline (particularly in the elderly populations), decrease monoamines involved in depression, reduce neuroplasticity, and increase the risk for falls, fractures, and episodes of confusion in the elderly populations. If the patient meets criteria for a Sedative/Hypnotic/Anxiolytic Use Disorder, recommendations for both non-pharmacological (rehabilitation/therapy) and pharmacological treatment (medication reduction/taper management) should be advised and documented [25, 26]. Within a medical hospital, consultation with case managers, social workers, and, if available, substance use counselors is recommended to discuss options with the patient and provide local resources, while also assisting with scheduling appts and/or program enrollment [2, 10, 13, 14].

There are no FDA-approved medications for the treatment of sedative/hypnotic/anxiolytic use disorder, with medications discussed above utilized primarily for withdrawal symptoms. Treatment of co-occurring anxiety, insomnia, and mood disorders is indicated to alleviate distress but also to assist with continued abstinence from benzodiazepines. Anxiolytic agents such as beta blockers (propranolol), pregabalin, and gabapentin can be utilized for residual anxiety. Insomnia can be treated with trazodone, doxepin, mirtazapine, hydroxyzine, diphenhydramine, doxylamine, or melatonin, along with improved sleep hygiene techniques. Anxiety or depressive disorders should be treated with serotonin reuptake inhibitors or other antidepressants [24].

3. Cannabis withdrawal and cannabis use disorder

Cannabis withdrawal can be characterized by the cessation of cannabis use that has been heavy and prolonged, with three or more signs and/or symptoms occurring within 1 week of cessation of cannabis, which include: irritability, anger, aggression, nervousness/anxiety, sleep difficulty, decreased appetite/weight loss, restlessness, depressed mood, abdominal pain, tremors, sweating, fever, chills, or headache. Cannabis cravings can occur during this time, leading to further use or relapse. Withdrawal symptoms typically begin between 24 and 48 hours from the last use, with withdrawal symptoms peaking from 2–6 days. The duration of withdrawal symptoms typically lasts 5–7 days; however, for heavy and chronic cannabis users, withdrawal symptoms may last up to 3 weeks. Insomnia, shakiness may occur first, then anxiety and irritability, followed by anger and aggression. In general, cannabis withdrawal does not carry an elevated risk of severe adverse outcomes; however, in combination with other substance abuse and medical co-morbidities, more serious complications from withdrawal may occur. Cannabis withdrawal in heavy cannabis users may more severely manifest and persist after ICU stabilization, leading to significant patient distress and requiring ongoing symptomatic treatment and observation [2, 27, 28].

Cannabis withdrawal evaluation is obtained through clinical evaluation, with a detailed substance use history and screening of co-occurring psychiatric symptoms to assist with symptomatic treatment and prediction of the withdrawal course [27]. Cannabis withdrawal treatment is primarily supportive, as there are no medications FDA-approved for cannabis withdrawal. While there are limited studies, with mixed results, Gabapentin (GABAergic modulation), Dronabinol, Nabilone, and Nabiximols (CB1 receptor agonists) have shown some efficacy for reducing cannabis withdrawal symptoms. These medications, however, did not assist with cravings or in the treatment of dependence. Many small studies involving multiple medications to include lithium, antidepressants, anticonvulsants, muscle relaxants, anxiolytics, antipsychotics, etc., have yielded no notable efficacy/benefit for withdrawal symptoms. For sleep disturbances related to withdrawal, there was some efficacy found in limited studies for mirtazapine and zolpidem within the first days of withdrawal; however, this treatment did not overall improve the withdrawal syndrome or relapse prevention. Quetiapine was found to have benefits in limited studies for appetite and sleep during withdrawal but worsened marijuana cravings and led to more cannabis use. There remains significant research needed to assist clinicians with more effective cannabis withdrawal management [29, 30].

Cannabis Use Disorder treatment involves primarily behavioral therapeutic interventions within outpatient or inpatient rehabilitation settings. Pharmacotherapy for Cannabis Use Disorder remains limited, with no FDA-approved medications to date; however, there is ongoing significant study into potential agents to assist with relapse prevention and craving. Patients admitted to the hospital with either concern for a cannabis use disorder or who have been admitted for/experienced cannabis withdrawal should be assessed for interest in cannabis cessation and to explore treatment goals. Patients should be screened for co-occurring psychiatric conditions that should be treated in conjunction with cannabis use disorder. Education regarding the risks of continued cannabis use on physical and mental health should be completed. Chronic heavy cannabis use has been associated with persistent decrements in neurocognitive performance (memory, learning), an increased risk of suicidal thinking/suicide, an increased risk of social anxiety disorder, depressive disorders, the development of psychosis/schizophrenia, and instigating mania in those with bipolar disorder. Cannabis Hyperemesis Syndrome is rare but severe and can occur with chronic and heavy cannabis use. This syndrome involves cyclical vomiting and severe abdominal pain, with nausea typically refractory to standard antiemetics. Capsaicin cream application, benzodiazepines, and even Haldol have been studied for use in persistent symptoms in small case studies. If the patient meets criteria for a Cannabis Use Disorder, recommendations for rehabilitation and therapeutic interventions should be advised and documented [31–35]. Within a medical hospital, consultation with case managers, social workers, and, if available, substance use counselors is recommended to discuss options with the patient and provide local resources, while also assisting with scheduling appts and/or program enrollment [2, 10, 13, 14].

There are no FDA-approved medications for the treatment of cannabis use disorder. Gabapentin had some benefit with limited studies of improving cannabis cravings, while Dronabinol, Nabiximols, and Nabilone have some evidence in their benefit for relapse prevention in combination with psychosocial treatments; however, substantial data remains limited. Some small studies with topiramate, oxytocin, NAC, and naltrexone have some positive data for assistance with relapse/abstinence; these remain unsubstantiated in most recent literature review. Associated treatment of residual anxiety, insomnia, or depression in concurrence with cannabis use disorder is recommended to assist in relieving distress and treating possible comorbid disorders [30, 36–38].

4. Hallucinogen withdrawal and hallucinogen use disorder

Hallucinogen withdrawal is not considered a separate phenomenon, as there is not typically a withdrawal syndrome after intoxication. However, persisting psychiatric symptoms are more common after intoxication, which may persist from days to weeks. It is important to remain vigilant for residual psychiatric symptoms post-ICU care to assist with the patient's distress and ensure the patient's ongoing safety. In some cases, psychiatric symptoms after hallucinogen use may become chronic, as seen in hallucinogen-persisting perception disorder. In this disorder, episodes of perceptual symptoms (hallucinations, intensified colors, afterimages, micropsia and macropsia, etc.) can persist intermittently long after cessation of hallucinogen use [2, 10, 39]. Some research indicates chronic Phencyclidine (PCP) use may produce withdrawal symptoms of drug craving, headaches, and sweating [40]. After the hallucinogen intoxication period, careful psychiatric symptoms screening should occur as significant anxiety, depression, manic-like symptoms, or psychosis may persist with or without suicidal or homicidal thinking. Hallucinogen-induced mood, anxiety, or psychotic disorders may manifest after use, and may require inpatient or ongoing outpatient psychiatric treatment, depending on severity and safety risk assessment. Persisting depressive symptoms, anxiety symptoms, or psychotic symptoms may require antidepressant or even antipsychotic use after psychiatric consultation. After acute intoxication, continued medical evaluation, primarily vital signs, laboratory evaluations, and cardiac monitoring may be required, especially in patients with acute and/or chronic medical complications [2, 10, 41].

There is minimal research data and clinical studies into the treatment of hallucinogen use disorder. There are no FDA-approved pharmacotherapies, and thus behavioral therapies remain the primary treatment. Patients admitted to the hospital with either concern for a hallucinogen/PCP use disorder or who have experienced/admitted for hallucinogen/PCP intoxication or withdrawal should be assessed for interest in hallucinogen/PCP cessation and explore treatment goals. Patients should be screened for co-occurring psychiatric conditions or other substance use disorders that should be treated in conjunction with the hallucinogen/PCP use disorder. Education regarding the risks of continued hallucinogen/PCP use on physical and mental health should be completed. Chronic use of hallucinogens/PCP can cause persistent neurotoxic effects impacting memory, speech, sleep, and psychiatric symptoms. Persisting anxiety, social withdrawal, depression, hallucinations, and other psychotic symptoms are the most common adverse effects from chronic hallucinogen use. Treatment of these persisting psychiatric symptoms requires the utilization of antidepressants, anxiolytic agents (avoid benzodiazepine use aside from intoxication treatment due to addiction risk), and antipsychotics.

5. Opioid withdrawal and opioid use disorder

Opioid withdrawal is considered one of the most distressing substance withdrawals. After acute stabilization in the ICU setting, continued observation and management of opioid withdrawal and opioid use disorder is imperative to avoid relapse and maintain abstinence. The acute phase of withdrawal may last 7–10 days. Management of opioid withdrawal involves symptomatic treatment, adjusting of hospital environment, and medication-assisted therapy. Patients who have been sedated or intubated in the ICU with fentanyl or have been receiving opioids for illness or injury with sudden cessation or decrease may then manifest withdrawal symptoms post-ICU stabilization, and thus awareness and vigilance regarding prior use history are important for withdrawal management.

An opioid withdrawal evaluation includes a diligent opioid use history (dose, duration, frequency of use), urine toxicology data, a complete blood count, a complete metabolic panel, consideration of HIV, Hep B and C tests, an ECG, a clinical evaluation of concurrent medical and psychiatric conditions, and an evaluation of current withdrawal symptoms. The Clinical Opioid Withdrawal Scale (COWS) protocol assists with evaluating the severity of opioid withdrawal by assessing resting pulse rate, GI upset, sweating, restlessness, tremor, yawning, anxiety or agitation, pupil size, bone/joint aches, gooseflesh skin, and running nose/tearing. The COWS score assists with detoxification medication management dosing and should be administered three to four times a day or more, depending on clinical severity [42–44].

Treatment involves detoxification with a long-acting opioid agonist or partial agonist, either methadone or buprenorphine, as a substitution for the patient's chronic opioid use occurring over several days to reduce and resolve withdrawal symptoms. The starting dose of either methadone or buprenorphine correlates to withdrawal severity and the patient's recent opioid use. For methadone substitution, on day 1 of withdrawal, a starting dose of 10–30 mg can be given. If withdrawal symptoms persist one hour after dosing, an additional 5–10 mg can be given. It is recommended that the total 24-hour methadone dose on the first day of detoxification should not exceed 40 mg. Continued evaluation of withdrawal symptoms should commence every 4–6 hours over the next 24 hours to assess a stable dosing of methadone with resolving or resolved withdrawal symptoms without oversedation. On days 2–4, the stabilized dose should be administered once daily, and after at least 24 hours of stability (resolved withdrawal symptoms), the dose can be tapered by 10–20% each day until discontinued. Methadone used for detoxification and dependence is utilized more effectively and frequently for individuals who require more than 60–70 mg of Methadone equivalent opioids due to its long elimination half-life.

For buprenorphine substitution, on day one of withdrawal symptoms, a 2–4 mg sublingual dosing can be administered, and if withdrawal symptoms persist after an hour, an additional 2–4 mg can be given. Additional dosing of 2–4 mg for continued withdrawal symptoms may be required after continued evaluation of withdrawal symptoms. Daily dosing typically reaches 12–16 mg for most patients. Continued withdrawal assessments over the next 24 hours should occur to assess a stable dosing of buprenorphine with resolving or resolved withdrawal symptoms without oversedation. On days 2–4, a stabilized buprenorphine dose should be administered, and after 24 hours of resolved withdrawal symptoms, the buprenorphine dose should be slowly tapered 10–20% daily until discontinued.

Symptomatic treatment for withdrawal symptoms is recommended to assist with the distress of withdrawal. Utilization of clonidine (while not FDA approved for withdrawal) has been helpful for mild withdrawal symptoms and can be given at 0.1–0.3 mg doses in three divided doses for the first day, typical max dosing 0.8–1.2 mg daily, with subsequent reduction in dose by 0.1–0.2 mg each day after for taper. Dosing typically is two to four times per day and tapered over several days to avoid rebound withdrawal or hypertension. Transdermal clonidine patches are available and can be effective. Careful monitoring of blood pressure is indicated and would be avoided in those with hypotension at baseline. Other medications utilized for symptomatic treatment of withdrawal include loperamide for diarrhea, nonsteroidal inflammatory agents for aches, antiemetics for nausea, and trazodone for insomnia. New studies and data are emerging regarding buprenorphine microinduction to assist with the transition of methadone or long-acting opioids to buprenorphine without requiring a period of withdrawal. This practice may assist patients who are on methadone for opioid withdrawal or maintenance therapy to transition to more readily accessible buprenorphine and avoid the risk of withdrawal/relapse more easily. Microinduction with buprenorphine involves lower dosing of buprenorphine sublingually at 0.25–2 mg while remaining on a long-acting opioid with gradual increases in dose to sustainable levels with then discontinuation of methadone or another long-acting opioid without taper. This practice still requires more extensive research and data from randomized and placebo-controlled trials but may be a viable option for safer utilization of opioid withdrawal and maintenance therapy in the future [2, 13, 14, 43, 45–48].

Management of Opioid Use Disorder involves both pharmacological and therapeutic interventions. Opioid maintenance therapy with a full or partial agonist is indicated for individuals meeting the criteria for opioid use disorder for one year or more. Not all patients with opioid withdrawal are abusing the substance, as certain opioids may be prescribed for chronic pain and then subsequently stopped suddenly due to acute medical decompensation or trauma. Chronic opioid users have higher rates of depression, with some studies indicating higher rates of post-traumatic stress disorder and personality disorders. Pharmacotherapy for Opioid Use Disorder involves FDA-approved maintenance opioid agonist or partial agonist treatment with methadone or buprenorphine, respectively. Intramuscular Naltrexone injections are also FDA-approved for Opioid Use Disorder. Initiation of pharmacotherapy for Opioid Use Disorder should always be discussed and considered in the hospital setting. Medication initiation for Opioid Use Disorder should be reserved for patients who are post-intubation with alert and clear mental status to ensure appropriate consent, the completion of an initial substance use evaluation, and due to the sedating nature of the pharmacotherapy intervention options.

Methadone maintenance treatment is regulated by federal and state licensure and is administered at a specific opioid treatment program by a specifically licensed physician. Hospitalized patients can be temporarily treated with methadone by hospital physicians without licensure while inpatient, however ongoing treatment and management after hospitalization must occur at a licensed methadone treatment program. Buprenorphine is an alternative and increasingly used partial mu agonist for opioid maintenance treatment. After hospitalization, buprenorphine administration can be done in office-based outpatient treatment programs with a certified provider in buprenorphine administration. Combination medications of buprenorphine and naloxone can be utilized to avoid misuse of buprenorphine as the additional naloxone is activated if buprenorphine is crushed in an attempt to snort/inject, naloxone's antagonist effect on the receptors nullifies any euphoria from the buprenorphine [47, 49, 50]. Naltrexone, a long-acting pure opioid antagonist can also be utilized for relapse prevention in opioid use disorder, with data indicating reduction in return to opioid use, reduced cravings, and increased treatment retention [50].

6. Stimulant withdrawal and stimulant use disorder

Stimulant withdrawal symptoms involve a typical "crash" period due to sudden catecholamine depletion, involving dysphoric mood development and at least two other symptoms to include fatigue, vivid dreams, insomnia or hypersomnia, increased appetite, and/or psychomotor agitation or retardation, all occurring within a few hours to several days after stimulant cessation. Other symptoms may include irritability, headache, profuse sweating, muscle cramps, stomach cramps, and intense drug craving later in the withdrawal period. Withdrawal peaks within two to four days after stimulant cessation, with resolution in roughly 1 week. Psychiatric symptoms typically are the most serious of stimulant withdrawal, with severe depression, and anhedonia, leading to suicidal thinking or suicide attempts; irritability and poor concentration may also manifest in withdrawal. Due to cocaine's half-life, its withdrawal is much more abrupt than methamphetamine however withdrawal symptomatology is remarkably similar if not identical to methamphetamine. Post-acute withdrawal syndrome includes residual psychiatric symptoms of depression, insomnia, anxiety, paranoia, and intense drug cravings that may last weeks to months and should be monitored carefully. After ICU stabilization, stimulant withdrawal must be carefully monitored, primarily in the context of the patient's safety and psychiatric symptomatology [2, 14, 16, 48, 51].

Treatment primarily involves symptomatic management and fostering a calm and quiet environment. There are no FDA-approved medications for stimulant withdrawal, and thus utilization of sleep aids for insomnia (trazodone, diphenhydramine), non-steroidal anti-inflammatory drugs for aches, and low-dose benzodiazepines for persisting and severe anxiety may be helpful over course of withdrawal duration. Residual psychotic symptoms, such as severe paranoia, delusions, or hallucinations should be treated with antipsychotic medications, with second-generation atypical antipsychotic formulations preferable due to their side effect profile. Careful evaluation of co-occurring psychiatric conditions is essential to adjust medication management and other interventions. Persisting psychiatric symptoms despite the resolution of physical manifestations of intoxication/withdrawal, such as residual depression, may require antidepressant treatment. Post-acute withdrawal symptoms may benefit from sedating antidepressants, antihistamines, melatonin, antipsychotics, and antihypertensives, depending on the residual symptom profile. Would avoid/caution use of sedative-hypnotics in post-acute withdrawal symptoms due to addiction risk. Persisting psychosis, suicidal, or homicidal thinking with resolving or improved withdrawal may require inpatient psychiatric admission and psychiatric consultation [51, 52].

The treatment of stimulant use disorder treatment at present primarily involves therapeutic interventions and psychosocial support. There is ongoing research in pharmacotherapies for stimulant use disorder, however, no FDA-approved treatments have been approved to date. Chronic stimulant use can lead to significant nutritional deficiencies/weight loss, headaches, tremors, dyskinesias, nasal septal perforation (with intranasal use), dental enamel corrosion (ingestion), ischemic colitis or other gastrointestinal complications, interstitial pneumonitis, renal ischemia, with increased risk for HIV and other infectious diseases, cardiovascular disease, cardiac arrhythmias, cardiomyopathy, and myocardial ischemia/infarction. Chronic stimulant use can impact multiple neurocognitive domains, disrupting working memory, attention, and executive functioning however can be reversible with cessation of use, and may lead to persistent psychosis remitting only after a prolonged period of abstinence.

Pharmacotherapy for Stimulant Use Disorder is without any FDA-approved options; however, there is ongoing research across many different medication classes to assist with cravings, sustain abstinence, and prevent relapse. Antidepressants such as desipramine, bupropion, and fluoxetine did not reduce cocaine dependence in trials but did assist with co-occurring mood symptoms. Non-SSRI antidepressants, such as mirtazapine, were found to better assist with mood symptoms than SSRIs. One small study found methamphetamine use reduction with mirtazapine but has not been replicated to date. Disulfiram utilization has yielded some positive results in the context of weeks of abstinence, but with low-quality evidence with small sample size trials. Antipsychotic utilization has been trialed for stimulant use disorder with no significant benefit for abstinence, although in some studies, antipsychotics did help with study retention. Anticonvulsant trials have yielded no significant or limited results, except for Topiramate, which has shown some positive results for continued abstinence and reduced drug cravings in smaller studies. The use of psychostimulants, to include modafinil, methylphenidate, dexamphetamine, and bupropion (trialed also in antidepressant categories), has yielded some positive but at times mixed results, particularly with modafinil and methylphenidate. Methylphenidate dosing has not shown adequate cocaine reduction in trials but has shown methamphetamine reductions in a few studies. Opioid agonist therapy involving buprenorphine-naloxone and methadone has been studied for concurrent opioid use disorder and stimulant use disorder, with methadone in small studies improving cocaine abstinence comparative to buprenorphine; however, there are no current comparative trials to placebo, and the evaluation of direct effect on cocaine use vs. opioid use has been difficult to ascertain. N-acetylcysteine (NAC) trials have yielded positive results in the reduction of cocaine cravings; however, findings from limited human data require further study. Bupropion-Naltrexone combination has found some positive results for methamphetamine type of stimulant use disorder. Other medications trialed for stimulant use disorder include butyrylcholinesterase, rivastigmine, doxazosin, and vigabatrin, with some positive results however with limited data; acupuncture has also been evaluated in stimulant reduction with no significant benefit in limited studies.

In general, off-label options for stimulant use disorder include topiramate, NAC, modafinil, methylphenidate, disulfiram, opioid agonists, bupropion-naltrexone, and mirtazapine; however, clear efficacy alone for stimulant use disorder is lacking and under continued study. These medications however may find more utility in co-occurring ADHD or depressive disorders with stimulant use disorder, or in combination for a concurrent additional substance use disorder [2, 10, 51, 53, 54].

7. Nicotine withdrawal and nicotine use disorder

Nicotine or tobacco withdrawal is similar for all nicotine related products. Criteria for withdrawal include daily use of tobacco for at least several weeks with associated abrupt cessation or reduction in amount of tobacco used subsequently leading to at least four signs or symptoms within 24 hours of cessation: irritability, frustration, anger, anxiety, poor concentration, increased appetite, restlessness, depressed mood, and insomnia. Other symptoms include intense tobacco craving, tension, decreased heart rate and blood pressure, decreased motor performance, and increased muscle tension. Withdrawal symptoms can initiate within 2 hours after the last use, peak around 48 hours from the last use, and diminish over several weeks. Psychiatric symptoms of depression, dysphoria, and anhedonia may last for several months. While tobacco withdrawal is not life-threatening, the withdrawal symptoms can cause significant distress and irritability post-ICU stabilization and will likely require assessment and treatment. Evaluation of Tobacco (nicotine) withdrawal should involve assessment of withdrawal symptoms, obtaining a detailed substance use history, and consideration of general laboratory evaluations to evaluate any co-occurring medical abnormalities. There are a few tobacco withdrawal scales to include the Minnesota Tobacco Withdrawal Scale and Wisconsin Smoking Withdrawal Scale that may be helpful to capture and monitor withdrawal symptoms [2, 35].

Nicotine (tobacco) withdrawal treatment involves nicotine replacement therapy which can double the chance of nicotine cessation. Nicotine replacement therapy (NRT) is FDA-approved for nicotine cessation to include tobacco (nicotine) withdrawal and tobacco use disorder. NRT should be reserved for individuals who are post-intubation and with clear mental status. Nicotine replacement therapy involves the initiation of replacement nicotine equivalent to the amount of tobacco previously utilized to resolve withdrawal symptoms. NRT has five formulations: nicotine gum, nicotine patch, nicotine inhaler, nicotine nasal spray, and a nicotine lozenge. Nicotine gum and lozenge dosages are 2 mg and 4 mg, with a maximum use of 24 pieces of gum (or lozenge) per day. Nicotine patches can be placed for 24 hours at doses of 7 mg, 14 mg, and 21 mg (>10 cigarettes per day) and a 16-hour dose at 15 mg. Nicotine inhalers utilize cartridges, from 6 to 16 cartridge availability per day. Nicotine nasal spray is a 1-mg droplet dose that can be used up to 30 to 40 times per day. Initiation of nicotine replacement can occur at any point in withdrawal or directly after tobacco cessation. Inclusion of NRT has been supported in research for hospitalized patients, as there are minimal and very mild adverse effects if occurring. Some data suggest utilization of both patch and another form of NRT is more effective at relieving withdrawal and cravings [2, 10, 13, 14, 48, 55, 56].

Nicotine use disorder treatment integrates both behavioral interventions and pharmacotherapy for the most effective route to abstinence. Pharmacotherapy for nicotine use disorder is more robust than other substance use disorders. FDA-approved medications include Bupropion SR, Varenicline, and nicotine replacement therapies. Nicotine Replacement Therapies (NRT) deliver nicotine concentrations at lower doses than tobacco products and rise more slowly thus reducing reinforcing effects. Nicotine gum and nicotine lozenges come in 2 mg or 4 mg doses with dose consideration based on number of cigarettes used per day. A 4 mg dose of gum or lozenge should be used if a patient utilizes 25 or more cigarettes per day or requires nicotine less than 30 min after awakening. Nicotine patches come in four different dosages, 7 mg, 14 mg, and 21 mg patches can be given every 24 hours and removed at night if causing anxiety/insomnia. A 15 mg patch can be utilized for 16 hours if preferred. A nicotine nasal spray uses 0.5 mg of nicotine per spray, with patients using one spray per nostril every 20–60 min for a maximum of 40 doses per day (80 sprays). A nicotine inhaler utilizes cartridges with nicotine concentrations, with an administration direction of 4 puffs/min for 20–30 min; 6–16 cartridges can be used per day.

Bupropion is an antidepressant, impacting norepinephrine and dopamine neurotransmitters and as a reuptake inhibitor increasing their release into the neuronal synapse. This increase in dopamine and norepinephrine mimics nicotine's effects on neurotransmission in the brain in an effort to reduce cravings and withdrawal effects. Dosing for Bupropion SR begins at 150 mg for three days and then 150 mg twice daily. Bupropion XL can be dosed at 150 mg once daily for three days and then increased to 300 mg once daily. A large meta-analysis evaluating over 60 randomized controlled studies found bupropion significantly increased long-term tobacco cessation. Other studies have found bupropion doubles the chances of smoking cessation versus placebo and may be beneficial in use with patients also diagnosed with depression. Bupropion is typically well tolerated outside of insomnia and dry mouth side effects, however, should be avoided in those with seizures or eating disorders as can lower the seizure threshold and suppress appetite [2, 28, 42, 57]. Varenicline is a nicotinic acetylcholine receptor partial agonist selective for the ventral tegmental area of the brain, which relieves nicotine cravings and withdrawal (due to partial stimulation of the receptor) and reduces reinforcing effects of nicotine use by blocking dopaminergic stimulation from tobacco products. Varenicline should be started

1 week prior to the tobacco quit date, with an uptitration dosing schedule of 0.5 mg in the morning for three days, then 0.5 mg twice per day for four days, and then 1 mg twice a day. Varenicline has been proven in multiple studies and large meta-analyses to greatly increase smoking cessation and sustain cessation with significant advantages in relapse prevention. Varenicline in comparison to bupropion was found to be superior in improving abstinence rates and is considered the most effective pharmacological intervention. Varenicline is typically well tolerated, however can cause nausea, sleep disturbance, and constipation. Varenicline and Bupropion do carry a black box warning for rare suicidal thinking in adolescents/young adults and can have some increase in depressed mood however the occurrence rates are quite low. Varenicline does have some possible increased risk for cardiovascular events, with careful monitoring of patients recommended [28, 55–58].

Combination medication therapy with NRT patch and gum/lozenge, along with NRT and bupropion, has proven efficacy in smoking cessation, especially in more severe tobacco (nicotine) addiction. Varenicline and NRT are also being studied with some initial data indicating effectiveness in cessation more than varenicline alone [28, 56]. Alternative options, not FDA-approved, include Nortriptyline which in small studies has had benefits for smoking cessation. Nortriptyline doses of 75–100 mg have been found effective for smoking cessation, with data from six randomized control trials indicating effectiveness for cessation compared to NRT or Bupropion. Clonidine historically has been utilized as an alternative for tobacco withdrawal and dependence by decreasing synaptic activity. Both treatments remain second-line due to limited research data and can cause more side effects. Studies on SSRIs have yielded no positive results. Ongoing clinical trials for novel tobacco cessation medications or interventions include Rimonabant—a cannabinoid receptor 1 antagonist of which has been found to demonstrate efficacy in smoking cessation but with concerning safety profile, Dopamine 3 antagonists, N-acetylcysteine, Cystisine, monoamine oxidase B inhibitors, aerosolized nicotine, nicotine vaccines, and repetitive Transcranial Magnetic Stimulation (in very early stages) [13, 28, 56].

Substance Use Disorder Treatment in the Outpatient Setting

After acute stabilization and acute withdrawal management, substance use disorder treatment almost always involves therapeutic interventions and for some substances associated pharmacotherapy. Both the psychological and pharmacological interventions may be initiated from multiple settings. Pharmacotherapy can be initiated during hospitalization, as noted above, however ongoing pharmacotherapy management and introduction of therapeutic treatments may occur through an inpatient rehabilitation program, intensive outpatient program, or outpatient addiction/substance abuse clinic. Rehabilitation aims to maintain motivation for abstinence, readjust lifestyle without the substance, enhance coping skills, facilitate self-change, and assist in relapse prevention. Recommendations for the level of rehabilitation involve the severity of the use disorder and patient interest. Criteria for rehabilitation placement from the American Society of Addiction Medicine include evaluation of acute intoxication or withdrawal potential, other medical conditions, other psychiatric or cognitive conditions, readiness to change, history of relapse, ongoing use, and the recovery/living environment. The levels of care for substance use disorders include outpatient (level one), intensive outpatient or partial hospitalization (level 2), and inpatient rehabilitation (level three) [39, 59]. Patients with severe withdrawal symptoms, long history of substance abuse, significant medical complications from the associated substance, and/or meeting criteria for moderate to severe substance use disorder would most benefit from an inpatient substance rehabilitation program. Inpatient rehabilitation is necessary for patients whose lives and social situations revolve around the substance, and who lack adequate vocational, social skills, and drug-free support networks to maintain abstinence in an outpatient setting. Patients who struggle with significant psychiatric diagnoses along with a substance use disorder, even if the substance use disorder is mild to moderate in severity, may also benefit from inpatient rehabilitation given the risk of acute psychiatric destabilization with substance use treatment.

Patients with mild to moderate substance withdrawal symptoms during hospitalization and who meet criteria for a substance use disorder with mild to moderate severity would most typically benefit from an intensive outpatient program (or partial hospitalization program) targeting substance use in an effort to prevent worsening of the use disorder and subsequent physical and mental health consequences. Intensive outpatient programs for substance abuse involve 3–5 days per week of 3–4 hours per day of intensive group and/or individual therapy targeting addiction treatment and may also include weekly medication management with a psychiatrist. Partial hospitalization programs are more intensive and are a direct step-down from an inpatient rehabilitation program, offering treatment five days per week with 4–8 hours of intensive group and/or individual therapy. Partial hospitalization programs or intensive outpatient programs are indicated for patients who need intensive rehabilitation care but have a higher probability of refraining from illicit substance use, have a history of relapse in post-rehabilitation settings, lack sufficient motivation for solely outpatient care, have severe co-occurring psychiatric illnesses, remain in high-risk environments with limited social support, or have failed outpatient management. Patients with Stimulant Use Disorder involving cocaine may be best treated in a more intensive outpatient setting from the beginning of treatment (at least twice per week appts) [13, 59].

Patients with mild withdrawal symptoms and meeting the mild severity of a SUD can typically benefit from outpatient substance use disorder programming in an outpatient clinic. An exception to the level of care algorithm involves nicotine use disorder. In the context of nicotine use disorder, inpatient rehabilitation alone has not been proven effective, with outpatient management found most beneficial and close clinical follow-up (1–3 days) after tobacco cessation recommended in the outpatient treatment setting [13]. Given the voluntary nature of SUD treatment (outside of court-ordered substance use treatment), patients may decline higher levels of rehabilitation and may be treated in an outpatient clinic even with recent intoxication and withdrawal symptoms with or without hospitalizations, with moderate or severe substance use disorder diagnoses. As patients complete inpatient rehabilitation and/or intensive outpatient/partial hospitalization programs, "graduation" to outpatient substance clinic care occurs for more long-term abstinence and relapse management. Substance use relapse is common in substance use disorders, and readmission to inpatient rehabilitation programs or intensive outpatient/partial hospitalization programs may occur throughout treatment.

The treatment of SUDs is a multi-faceted approach to treating both psychological and physiological symptoms related to continued dependence on the substance and avoidance of withdrawal symptoms. Certain SUDs require more frequent and structured outpatient care management for pharmacotherapy, while all SUDs as a whole benefit from regular utilization of counseling and therapeutic interventions throughout treatment and abstinence. It is also important to always evaluate and treat co-occurring psychiatric disorders in association with a substance use disorder, as in most cases, each disorder can exacerbate the condition of the other. Opioid Use Disorder requires a more intensive and structured outpatient medical management due to evidence-based interventions of opioid replacement and assisted therapy. Given the risks of scheduled opioids for purposes of maintaining abstinence, outpatient care for Opioid Use Disorder requires daily (methadone) or weekly (buprenorphine) outpatient office visits at implementation and for ongoing treatment (buprenorphine can be moved to monthly after continued stability over several months). This pharmacotherapy treatment is recommended to be paired with ongoing substance abuse counseling, whether that is individual or group with additional 12-step programming or self-help interventions; these interventions should be regular and consistent (i.e., daily to weekly). Opioid Use Disorder requires both regular and consistent pharmacotherapy and behavioral intervention for sustained abstinence.

Alcohol use disorder, sedative/hypnotic/anxiolytic use disorder, and nicotine use disorder also require more regular outpatient visits and medical management but typically are not as intensive in the context of pharmacotherapy. Initiation of anti-craving agents for alcohol use disorder, nicotine replacement therapy for nicotine use disorder, and benzodiazepine (or other sedative/hypnotic/anxiolytics) taper for sedative/hypnotic/anxiolytic use disorder, benzodiazepine type, require closer monitoring weekly or every few weeks at initiation, but can be maintained monthly with continued stability/abstinence. Therapeutic interventions are recommended to be paired with pharmacotherapy to include substance abuse counseling (individual or group) with additional 12-step programming or self-help interventions; these interventions should be regular and consistent (i.e., daily to weekly).

Cannabis, Stimulant, and Hallucinogen/Phencyclidine use disorders do not currently have FDA-approved pharmacotherapy for treatment; however, clinical studies are ongoing, and some treatments may be utilized off-label. Most medical management for the associated SUD is limited and primarily involves symptom management from either withdrawal states or persisting physical or psychiatric symptoms after intoxication or withdrawal. Outpatient appointments, unless utilizing off-label treatment, depend on symptom management and vary based upon symptom severity. Stimulant Use Disorder has more data to suggest trial of off-label medication treatments, and thus outpatient medical management may be more frequent. Therapeutic interventions, however, remain recommended for these disorders (with limited data on the type of treatment for hallucinogen use disorder) to include substance abuse counseling (individual or group) with additional self-help or associated 12-step programming if available. Therapy interventions should remain regular and consistent (daily or weekly, ideally) for continued abstinence.

Conclusion

SUDs greatly impact our health care system and, more importantly, cause significant distress and dysfunction for our patients. The evaluation and treatment of intoxication, withdrawal, and a substance use disorder in a timely and efficient manner can greatly impact both the acute and chronic effects of the substance. SUD treatment in a hospital setting should focus not only on acute stabilization and symptom management but also on the initiation of education and the implementation of evidence-based substance use disorder interventions in an effort to begin rehabilitation and recovery.

References

1. American Psychiatric Association. Diagnostic and statistical manual of mental disorders. 5th ed. American Psychiatric Publishing; 2013.
2. De La Garza R, Haile C, Kosten T, Newton T. Substance-related and addictive disorders. In: Hales R; Robers, L; Yudofsky, S (Eds.), Textbook of psychiatry, DSM- 5 Edition, 6th ed, p. 735–803). The American Psychiatric Publishing; 2014.
3. Koob GF, Volkow ND. Neurobiology of addiction: a neurocircuitry analysis. Lancet Psychiatry. 2016;3(8):760–73. https://doi.org/10.1016/S2215-0366(16)00104-8.
4. Volkow ND, Wang GJ, Fowler JS, Tomasi D. Addiction circuitry in the human brain. Annu Rev Pharmacol Toxicol. 2012;52:321–36. https://doi.org/10.1146/annurev-pharmtox-010611-134625.
5. The ASAM clinical practice guideline on alcohol withdrawal management. J Addic Med;14(3S):1–72, May/June 2020. https://doi.org/10.1097/ADM.0000000000000668.
6. Ballard HS. The hematological complications of alcoholism. Alcohol Health Res World. 1997;21(1):42–52.
7. Lewis MJ. Alcoholism and nutrition: a review of vitamin supplementation and treatment. Curr Opin Clin Nutr Metab Care. 2020;23(2):138–44. https://doi.org/10.1097/MCO.0000000000000622.
8. Andresen-Streichert H, Müller A, Glahn A, Skopp G, Sterneck M. Alcohol biomarkers in clinical and forensic contexts. Deutsches Arzteblatt International. 2018;115(18):309–15. https://doi.org/10.3238/arztebl.2018.0309.
9. Clinical Institute Withdrawal Assessment, of Alcohol Scale Revised (2001). American Society of Addiction Medicine. ciwa-ar.pdf (va.gov).
10. Ruiz P, Sadock B, Sadock V. Substance use and addictive disorders. Kaplan & Sadock's synopsis of psychiatry, behavioral sciences/clinical psychiatry, Eleventh Edition. Walters Kluwer; 2015. p. 616–684.

11. Sachdeva A, Choudhary M, Chandra M. Alcohol withdrawal syndrome: benzodiazepines and beyond. J Clin Diagn Res. 2015;9(9):VE01–7. https://doi.org/10.7860/JCDR/2015/13407.6538.
12. Stahl SM. Stahl's essential psychopharmacology: neuroscientific basis and practical applications. 7th ed. Cambridge University Press; 2014.
13. Treating Substance use Disorders: a quick reference guide. American Psychiatric Association, Steering Committee on Practice Guidelines. Based on practice guideline for the treatment of patients with substance use disorders, Second Edition. Originally published 2006. https://psychiatryonline.org/pb/assets/raw/sitewide/practice_guidelines/guidelines/substanceuse-guide.pdf
14. McGovern MP, Carroll KM. Evidence-based practices for substance use disorders. Psychiatr Clin North Am. 2003;26(4):991–1010. https://doi.org/10.1016/s0193-953x(03)00073-x.
15. Krimpuri R, Youngs C, Emerman C. Initiation of medication for alcohol use disorder for inpatients with alcohol withdrawal syndromes. J Stud Alcohol Drugs. 2023;84(2):293. https://doi.org/10.15288/jsad.22-00219. Epub 2022 Nov 7
16. Clinical guidelines for withdrawal management and treatment of drug dependence in closed settings. Geneva: World Health Organization; 2009. 4, Withdrawal Management. Available from: https://www.ncbi.nlm.nih.gov/books/NBK310652/
17. Park T. Benzodiazepine use disorder. In: UpToDate, Stein M, editor. Wolters Kluwer. Accessed 04 Dec 2023.
18. Soyka M. Treatment of benzodiazepine dependence. N Engl J Med. 2017;376(12):1147–57. https://doi.org/10.1056/NEJMra1611832.
19. Benzodiazepine withdrawal scale. University of North Carolina Eshelman School of Pharmacy. 1989. https://deprescribe.web.unc.edu/wp-content/uploads/sites/20194/2019/08/CIWA-B-Benzodiazepine-Withdrawal-Scale.pdf
20. Busto UE, Sykora K, Sellers EM. A clinical scale to assess benzodiazepine withdrawal. J Clin Psychopharmacol. 1989;9(6):412–6.
21. Bounds CG, Nelson VL. Benzodiazepines. [Updated 2023 Jan 7]. In: StatPearls [Internet]. Treasure Island (FL): StatPearls Publishing; 2023 Jan-. Available from: https://www.ncbi.nlm.nih.gov/books/NBK470159/
22. Edinoff AN, Nix CA, Hollier J, Sagrera CE, Delacroix BM, Abubakar T, Cornett EM, Kaye AM, Kaye AD. Benzodiazepines: uses, dangers, and clinical considerations. Neurol Int. 2021;13(4):594–607. https://doi.org/10.3390/neurolint13040059.
23. Gallo AT, Hulse G. Pharmacological uses of flumazenil in benzodiazepine use disorders: a systematic review of limited data. J Psychopharmacol (Oxford, England). 2021;35(3):211–20. https://doi.org/10.1177/0269881120981390.
24. Lader M, Kyriacou A. Withdrawing benzodiazepines in patients with anxiety disorders. Curr Psychiatry Rep. 2016;18:8. https://doi.org/10.1007/s11920-015-0642-5,
25. Lim, Bryant[a]; Sproule, Beth A.[b,,c]; Zahra, Zarin[a]; Sunderji, Nadiya[d]; Kennedy, Sidney H.[a,,e,,f]; Rizvi, Sakina J.[a,,e,,f]. Understanding the effects of chronic benzodiazepine use in depression: a focus on neuropharmacology. Int Clin Psychopharmacol;35(5):243–253, September 2020. https://doi.org/10.1097/YIC.0000000000000316.
26. Markota M, Rummans T, Bostwick J, Lapid M. Benzodiazepine use in older adults: dangers, management, and alternative therapies. Mayo Clin Proc. 2016;91(11):1632–9. https://doi.org/10.1016/j.mayocp.2016.07.024.
27. Connor JP, Stjepanović D, Budney AJ, Le Foll B, Hall WD. Clinical management of cannabis withdrawal. Addiction. 2022;117(7):2075–95. https://doi.org/10.1111/add.15743.
28. Polosa R, Benowitz NL. Treatment of nicotine addiction: present therapeutic options and pipeline developments. Trends Pharmacol Sci. 2011;32(5):281–9. https://doi.org/10.1016/j.tips.2010.12.008.
29. Bonnet U, Preuss UW. The cannabis withdrawal syndrome: current insights. Subst Abus Rehabil. 2017;8:9–37. https://doi.org/10.2147/SAR.S109576.
30. Brezing CA, Levin FR. The current state of pharmacological treatments for cannabis use disorder and withdrawal. Neuropsychopharmacology Off Public Am Coll Neuropsychopharmacology. 2018;43(1):173–94. https://doi.org/10.1038/npp.2017.212.

31. Chu F, Cascella M. Cannabinoid hyperemesis syndrome. [Updated 2023 Jul 3]. In: StatPearls [Internet]. Treasure Island (FL): StatPearls Publishing; 2023 Jan-. Available from: https://www.ncbi.nlm.nih.gov/books/NBK549915/
32. Health Affects of Marijuana. National Center for Injury Prevention and Control, Centers for Disease Control and Prevention. 2021. https://www.cdc.gov/marijuana/health-effects/index.html
33. Memedovich KA, Dowsett LE, Spackman E, Noseworthy T, Clement F. The adverse health effects and harms related to marijuana use: an overview review. CMAJ Open. 2018;6(3):E339–46. https://doi.org/10.9778/cmajo.20180023.
34. National Academies of Sciences, Engineering, and Medicine; Health and Medicine Division; Board on Population Health and Public Health Practice; Committee on the Health Effects of Marijuana: An Evidence Review and Research Agenda. The Health Effects of Cannabis and Cannabinoids: The Current State of Evidence and Recommendations for Research. Washington (DC): National Academies Press (US); 2017 Jan 12. 12, Mental Health. Available from: https://www.ncbi.nlm.nih.gov/books/NBK425748/
35. Ross JM, Ellingson JM, Frieser MJ, Corley RC, Hopfer CJ, Stallings MC, Wadsworth SJ, Reynolds CA, Hewitt JK. The effects of cannabis use on physical health: a co-twin control study. Drug Alcohol Depend. 2022;230:109200. https://doi.org/10.1016/j.drugalcdep.2021.109200.
36. Bahji A, Meyyappan AC, Hawken ER, Tibbo PG. Pharmacotherapies for cannabis use disorder: a systematic review and network meta-analysis. Int J Drug Policy. 2021;97:103295. https://doi.org/10.1016/j.drugpo.2021.103295.
37. Connor JP, Stjepanović D, Le Foll B, Hoch E, Budney AJ, Hall WD. Cannabis use and cannabis use disorder. Nat Rev Dis Primers. 2021;7(1):16. https://doi.org/10.1038/s41572-021-00247-4.
38. Sabioni P, Le Foll B. Psychosocial and pharmacological interventions for the treatment of cannabis use disorder. Focus Psychiat. 2019;17:163–8. https://doi.org/10.1176/appi.focus.17202.
39. Detoxification and Substance Abuse Treatment [Internet]. Rockville (MD): Substance Abuse and Mental Health Services Administration (US); 2006. (Treatment Improvement Protocol (TIP) Series, No. 45.) 2 Settings, Levels of Care, and Patient Placement. Available from: https://www.ncbi.nlm.nih.gov/books/NBK64109/
40. Hallucinogens and Dissociative Drugs, Research Report Series. 2014. National Institute on Drug Abuse. National Institute of Health. https://nida.nih.gov/sites/default/files/rrhalluc.pdf
41. Journey JD, Bentley TP. Phencyclidine toxicity. [Updated 2023 Sep 4]. In: StatPearls [Internet]. Treasure Island (FL): StatPearls Publishing; 2023 Jan-. Available from: https://www.ncbi.nlm.nih.gov/books/NBK507865/
42. Moore, Dorothy J. DNP, CCRN, FNP-C. A quick guide to the Clinical Opiate Withdrawal Scale. Nursing Made Incredibly Easy! 18(3):6–9, May/June 2020. https://doi.org/10.1097/01.NME.0000658212.31416.a5.
43. Shah M, Huecker MR. Opioid withdrawal. [Updated 2023 Jul 21]. In: StatPearls [Internet]. Treasure Island (FL): StatPearls Publishing; 2023 Jan-. Available from: https://www.ncbi.nlm.nih.gov/books/NBK526012/
44. Wesson DR, Ling W. The clinical opiate withdrawal scale (COWS). J Psychoactive Drugs. 2003;35(2):253–9. https://doi.org/10.1080/02791072.2003.10400007). Clinical Opiate Withdrawl Scale (nih.gov)
45. De Aquino JP, Parida S, Sofuoglu M. The pharmacology of buprenorphine microinduction for opioid use disorder. Clin Drug Investig. 2021;41(5):425–36. https://doi.org/10.1007/s40261-021-01032-7.
46. Robbins J, Englander H, Gregg J. Buprenorphine microdose induction for the management of prescription opioid dependence. J Am Board Family Med. 2021;34(Supplement):S141–6. https://doi.org/10.3122/jabfm.2021.S1.200236.
47. The ASAM National Practice Guideline for the Use of Medications in the Treatment of Addiction Involving Opioid Use (2015). Available at: http://www.asam.org/docs/default-source/practicesupport/guidelines-and-consensus-docs/national-practice-guideline.pdf. Accessed 7Dec 2023. https://www.samhsa.gov/sites/default/files/sites/default/files/opioid-addiction-asam-use-of-medications-in-treatment.pdf

48. Weaver M. Substance-related disorders. In: Levenson J, editor. Textbook of psychosomatic medicine and consultation-liaison psychiatry. 3rd ed. The American Psychiatric Association Publishing; 2019. p. 435–62.
49. Kumar R, Viswanath O, Saadabadi A. Buprenorphine. [Updated 2023 Nov 30]. In: StatPearls [Internet]. Treasure Island (FL): StatPearls Publishing; 2023 Jan-. Available from: https://www.ncbi.nlm.nih.gov/books/NBK459126/
50. Mosel S. Suboxone: Uses, Side Effects & Addiction. Thomas, S (Ed.), American Addiction Centers. 2023. https://americanaddictioncenters.org/suboxone
51. ASAM AAP Clinical Practice Guideline on the Management of Stimulant Use Disorder (2023). American Society of Addiction Medicine. https://downloads.asam.org/sitefinity-production-blobs/docs/default-source/quality-science/stud_guideline_document_final.pdf?sfvrsn=71094b38_1
52. Treatment for Stimulant Use Disorders: Updated 2021 [Internet]. Rockville (MD): Substance Abuse and Mental Health Services Administration (US); 1999. (Treatment Improvement Protocol (TIP) Series, No. 33.) Chapter 3—Medical aspects of stimulant use disorders. Available from: https://www.ncbi.nlm.nih.gov/books/NBK576550/
53. Liu MT. Pharmacotherapy treatment of stimulant use disorder. Mental Health Clin. 2021;11(6):347–57. https://doi.org/10.9740/mhc.2021.11.347.
54. Park T, Haning W. Stimulant use disorders. Child Adolesc Psychiatr Clin N Am. 2016;25(3):461–71. https://doi.org/10.1016/j.chc.2016.02.004.
55. Integrating tobacco use disorder interventions in addiction treatment: a guide for addiction treatment clinicians and programs. 2023. American Society of Addiction Medicine. https://sitefinitystorage.blob.core.windows.net/sitefinity-production-blobs/docs/default-source/guidelines/tobacco-guide.pdf?sfvrsn=c8d48d75_3%20onclick=%E2%80%9D_gaq.push(%5b%E2%80%98_trackEvent%E2%80%99,%E2%80%99Download%E2%80%99,%E2%80%99PDF%E2%80%99,this.href%5d);%E2%80%9D
56. NIDA. 2021, April 12. What are treatments for tobacco dependence? Retrieved from https://nida.nih.gov/publications/research-reports/tobacco-nicotine-e-cigarettes/what-are-treatments-tobacco-dependence on 2024, January 5.
57. Ziedonis D, Das S, Larkin C. Tobacco use disorder and treatment: new challenges and opportunities. Dialogues Clin Neurosci. 2017;19(3):271–80. https://doi.org/10.31887/DCNS.2017.19.3/dziedonis.
58. Chelladurai Y, Singh S. Varenicline and cardiovascular adverse events: a perspective review. Therap Adv Drug Saf. 2014;5(4):167–72. https://doi.org/10.1177/2042098614530421.
59. Padwa, Howard PhD; Mark, Tami L. PhD; Wondimu, Betselot BS. What's in an "ASAM-based Assessment?" Variations in assessment and level of care determination in systems required to use ASAM patient placement criteria. J Addict Med. 2022;16(1):18–26. https://doi.org/10.1097/ADM.0000000000000804.

Index

K. Karamchandani, J. E. Grant (eds.), *Substance Use Disorders in Adult Critically Ill Patients*, https://doi.org/10.1007/978-3-031-67069-5

T

W

Printed by Printforce, the Netherlar